dysiexia

Insights into the hidden disability in and out of the workplace

Dr Shae Marie Wissell

KMD
BOOKS

A catalogue record for this
work is available from the
National Library of Australia

NATIONAL
LIBRARY
OF AUSTRALIA

National Library of Australia Catalogue-in-Publication data:
Dyslexia / Shae Wissell

ISBN:

In loving memory of my mum
Victoria Wissell,
Educator, Leader, grandmother, wife, sister and dear friend
to many.
To my beautiful mother, there are no words, but I know you
are always by my side,
I'm finally here ma I made it.
I promised you I would!

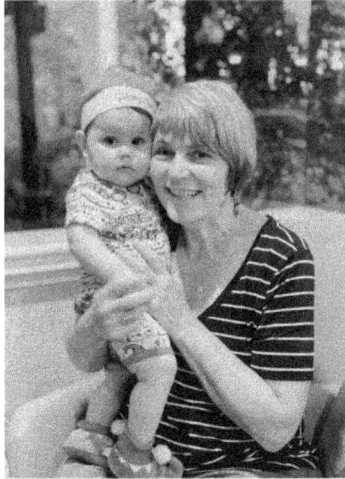

Dr Shae Marie Wissell

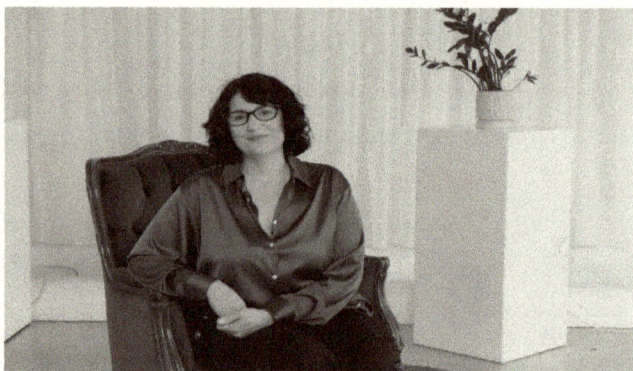

Dr Shae Marie Wissell is a respected thought leader, researcher and international award-winning advocate for adults with dyslexia and other neurodivergences. She is a certified practising speech pathologist with a Master of Public Health and Health Administration and a Doctor of Public Health. A seasoned entrepreneur, Shae has extensive experience in health, not-for-profit, and social enterprise industries, and she uses her business acumen to create successful ventures. She brings a wealth of expertise to her work, running her own successful businesses as the director of **re:think dyslexia** and founder of the Dear Dyslexic Foundation, Dyslexia Research Centre its partnering charity. Shae leverages her diverse skillset and lived experiences of neurodivergence to offer valuable coaching, advocacy, research and workforce solutions to individuals, entrepreneurs and organisations looking to take their lives and businesses to the next level.

Shae's research centres on the lived experiences of adults with dyslexia in Australia. Her work explores the social inequalities individuals with dyslexia may face across healthcare, education, employment, interpersonal relationships, and social and emotional well-being. Shae has published locally and internationally on work experiences, mental health, and well-being.

Shae is an accomplished workplace advisor who offers consulting, learning, and development programs that provide invaluable guidance to businesses seeking to create more inclusive workplaces through **re:think dyslexia.** Her expertise in neurodivergence has been instrumental in shaping workplace policies and training programs that foster greater diversity, equity and inclusion and helping organisations unlock the full potential of their neurodiverse employees. Through her innovative approaches to advocacy and education, Shae is creating a brighter future for individuals with dyslexia and other neurodivergences, while helping educators and workplaces thrive in an increasingly competitive marketplace.

In addition to her research, Shae has won numerous international and national awards. Most recently she was Highly Commended for her research with the Learning Difficulties Australia Tertiary Awards and was recognised in the U.K Corporate Vision Awards for Best Dyslexia Coaching Program. Shae is a confident public speaker, host of the Dear Dyslexic and the Hobo CEO podcast series, and published author. Her debut book, "The Hobo CEO: A Year in the Life of a Dyslexic Social Entrepreneur," reached the top spot on Amazon's bestseller list. With her unique blend of personal and professional expertise, Shae is seen as an asset to the dyslexia community and beyond.

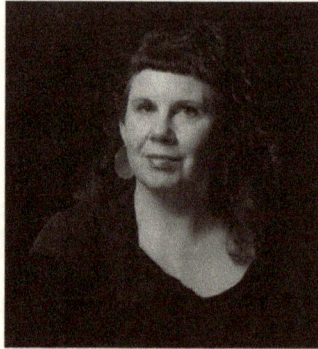

The book cover

The book cover was created by Kim Percy an artist, designer, PhD student and proud dyslexic. The cover draws inspiration from the fact that 1 in 10 people are dyslexic, symbolised by a red figure, standing tall among a sea of grey. The textures within the figures are taken from Kim's paintings, featuring overlapping handwriting that reflects the challenges dyslexics often face with written language. The concentric circles behind the figures evoke a target, focusing attention, ripples in a pond symbolising the spread of influence, and the rings of time spiralling outward. The blocky, difficult-to-read title font mirrors the struggles many dyslexics encounter with reading and the complexity of the word 'dyslexia'—with 'dys' meaning difficulty and 'lexia' referring to words or reading. The cover also highlights the strengths of dyslexia, including visual-spatial aware-ness, thinking in pictures, and strong visual communication. Kim is currently completing her PhD in visual art and dyslexia.

Contents

Acknowledgement... xii

Prologue xii
Background to the research xx
Publications from this research xxiii

PART ONE: The Journey into Adulthood................................1
Chater One: Dyslexia..3
1.1. What is dyslexia 4
1.2. Causation...8
1.2.1. Brain architecture, the neurobiological basis of dyslexia 8
1.3. The influence of genetics 9
1.4. Prevalence 10
1.5. Dyslexia and co-occurring difficulties...........................11
1.5.1. Dyslexia and dyscalculia 11
1.5.2. Dyslexia and dysgraphia 12
1.5.3. Dyslexia and dyspraxia 12
1.5.4. Dyslexia and Autism..13
1.5.5. Dyslexia and Attention-deficit/hyperactivity disorder 13
1.5.6. Dyslexia and Developmental Language Disorder 14

1.5.7. Dyslexia and social and emotional well-being 15
1.6. Conclusions...16

Chapter 2: Dyslexia, labels and models...21
2.1. Medical model 22
2.2. Social Model of Disability 24
2.3. Neurodivergence is more than Autism and ADHD 25
2.4. Bronfenbrenner Ecological Model..28
2.5. Intersectionality 29
2.6. Conclusion 32

Chapter 3: The dyslexic journey to the workplace through the lens
of Bronfenbrenner 35
3.1. The macrosystem 36
   3.1.1. Political systems 37
   3.1.2. Legal influences 39
3.2. The exosystem...48
   3.2.1. Communities..49
      3.2.1.1. Diagnosing Dyslexia 49
      3.2.1.2. Who can diagnose us and how 52
      3.2.1.3. Is a diagnosis important?...54
      3.2.1.4. Access to mental health services 56
   3.2.2. Societal influences 58
      3.2.2.1. Ableism and Labels 58
      3.2.2.2. High profile dyslexics and the Dyslexia 'Superpower'
      Narrative 60
3.3. The mesosystem 67
   3.3.1. Negative childhood experiences 67
   3.3.2. Education and qualifications 69
   3.3.3. Relationships and social connections 71

3.3.4. Family support and other relationships.................................75

3.3.5. The pros and cons of technology when communicating ..80

3.4. Conclusion 81

3.5. The microsystem 83

3.5.1. Trauma and Post Traumatic Stress Syndrome Disorder ...85

3.5.2. Self-concept 87

3.5.3. Mental health and well-being 88

3.5.4. Conclusion..91

Part Two: The Journey into the workplace:a dyslexic perspective........97

Chapter 4: Dyslexic employee profile 99

4.1. Dyslexia Difficulties 99

4.1.1. Literacy skills..101

4.1.1.1.Reading 101

4.1.1.2. Writing Skills...102

4.1.1.3. Numerous Skills...103

4.2. Executive functioning difficulties for dyslexics....................104

4.3. Verbal communication 105

4.4. Cognitive overload equals mental fatigue 106

4.5. Coping strategies: some call masking, some call passing 108

4.6. Lack of awareness and understanding..............................111

4.7. Dyslexia Strengths: personal resources 112

4.8. Conclusion 115

Chapter 5: Do you see me, to disclose or not to disclose 118

5.1. To Disclose or not to Disclose - that is the question. 119

5.2. How to disclose my dyslexia to my manager and or employer
....122

5.3.How to talk to a team member who you think might be dyslexic 125

5.4. Conclusion 129

Chapter 6: Unravelling Workplace Challenges: Recognising Internal Barriers 135

6.1. ...Transitioning into the workplace from school - how we can support young adults. 137

6.2. Recruitment and onboarding practices...................................144

6.2.1.Accessible role advertising:.......................................147

6.2.2.Accessible Job Descriptions:.....................................147

6.2.3.Flexible Application Process:....................................148

6.2.4. Clear Communication: 148

6.2.5. Psychometric assessments 149

6.2.6. Interview procedures 150

6.3. Retention 152

6.4. Career progression 156

6.5. Conclusion 157

6.6. Conclusion: 165

Chapter 7: Workplace well-being and burnout 169

7.1. Psychological safety in the workplace 170

7.2. Burnout...172

7.3.Dyslexia and the Job Demands Resource Model of Burnout (JD-R Model) 173

7.4. Dyslexia and work-related psychological distress and burnout..176

7.5.Mitigating Psychosocial Hazards and Burnout for Dyslexic Individuals..178

7.6. Conclusion 180

Chapter 8: Setting dyslexic talent up for success in the workplace..193

8.1. The role of the dyslexic employee 194

8.2. The role of the manager and leadership team 196

8.3. The role of the organisation 199

8.4. Reframing workplaces using Universal design principles 203

8.5. What are Workplace accommodations?....................................204

8.6.Assistive technology...205

8.7. Non-tech support...208

8.8. The role of mentors and coaching employees with dyslexia ..210

8.9. Australian funding support 213

8.9.1. What is the Employment Assistance Fund...................214

8.9.2. What is JobAccess?...214

8.10. Mental health support in the workplace 215

8.11. Conclusion 217

Chapter 9: Looking after yourself as a dyslexic adult 222

Chapter 10: The Dyslexic Golden Threads that create the tapestry of life 230

10.1. The way forward 231

   10.1.1. Community awareness and public health messaging.....231

   10.1.2. Improved access to appropriate assessments and early intervention..232

   10.1.3. mproved social and emotional well-being of dyslexic adults..233

   10.1.4. Improve workplace practices through training 234

   10.1.5. Streamlined and the states and government brought into alignment with access to health care, education and employment...235

   10.1.6. Increase in data collection and surveillance 236

   10.1.7. Future research...236

   10.1.8. A proactive approach 237

Glossary of Terms...240

References 247

Acknowledgement

It's hard to acknowledge everyone who has supported me through this crazy journey, from family to friends to complete strangers. It is the gift of time that people have offered so generously even though they have busy lives, competing priorities and families of their own. These people have offered guidance, support and mentorship. I set out on this journey to prove something to myself; that I was smart and intelligent. There was something inside of me determined to complete a doctorate. I discovered on this journey how determined, persistence and resilient I really am - all very strong dyslexic traits. There have been some significant difficult personal times when I thought I wouldn't get to the end of this chapter of my life that I have so carefully and passionately carved. It is that passion that has kept me going, as well as the continuing injustice I see so many people with dyslexia face daily. That injustice and an insatiable drive for social equity and justice has pushed me through the dark times of self-doubt, questioning and personal struggles of having dyslexia. This has been one of the hardest journeys of self-discovery I've been on. But the sum of what I hope to achieve is greater than me, and I hope this thesis gives a voice to those who participated in this research. I hope that, with these voices and the voices of many others, we can start to create systemic changes for young people and adults with dyslexia in Australia. For far too long we have been silenced, we have not had a voice, we have been spoken for and about, but until now, we have not been at the table or part of the conversation. I hope this thesis will start to give a voice to the silenced, the unseen, the ignored, the ill-treated, the 1 in 10 Australians who, like me, have dyslexia.

It has been an honour and privilege to be able to bring these stories to life through this research and, for the first time in Australia, have research that starts to paint a picture of what life is truly like for those with dyslexia. It's a hard story to share. There have been many tears in hearing and representing these through our research. Through the sharing of these stories of people with dyslexia in Australia and the ongoing support of my family, friends, dyslexic community and supervisors, I have reached my desired destination in completing this book. To my family, my biggest supporters (full of neurodiversity) - they have run the hard race, stood by my side, edited my work, never once questioned my hopes and dreams, and said go for it. Thank you to my aunty, Leanne Di Stefano, who has supported my doctoral journey, editing and reviewing my work and spending countless hours going through my thoughts and ideas with me.

To my beautiful mum, Victoria, who is no longer with us - without her ongoing support, love, and unwavering belief in me, I would never have completed secondary school, let alone have an undergraduate degree, two Masters, and now a Doctorate. Not only did she help by editing all my work through my life, but she also held me in her arms and cared for me in my darkest days. I am eternally thankful the universe chose me to be your daughter.

To my kind, caring partner, who cooked and cleaned, danced with me, held me and cried with me, encouraged me when I said I wanted to give this up because it was too hard, I couldn't do it. He has tended to our beautiful family, while I worked on making my dream a reality.

To the participants - I hope I have made you proud of being part of Australian first research. I am proud of the work we have achieved. This work is for them – the greater sum of me.

Last, but not least, I would like to acknowledge the dyslexic community and all those who have struggled to reach their dreams and to see their full potential. This research, all the blood, sweat and tears, are for you. I hope you can see that you can dream, and those dreams can come true. It's not easy, I won't lie, and sometimes our dreams are adjusted, but we can all reach our full potential, whatever that means to you.

This book is an original contribution and Australian-first research developed with oversight from my supervisors:

- Dr Leila Karimi, A/Professor of Organisational Psychology; Accredited Statistician, Assistant Associate Dean-Applied health (HoD Psychology Department) Applied Health, Psychology School of Health and Biomedical Sciences RMIT,
- Dr Tanya Serry Associate Professor Speech Pathologist, School of Education, La Trobe University
- Dr Lisa Furlong, La Trobe University
- Dr Judith Hudson, College of Arts, Law and Education -CALE, School of Education University of Tasmania. They were also co-authors of the three journal papers published through the research conducted.

Thank you for your ongoing support and guidance through my research journey.

This book brings new learnings about the lived-experiences, in adulthood, of Australians with Dyslexia. Through research undertaken, this book takes you on a journey that uncovers the entrenched ignorance of Dyslexia across the social determinants of health; education, employment, social and emotional well-being, as well as a pathway that can lead to inferior quality of life outcomes for adults who live with dyslexia throughout their lifetime. This research and book are a response to the need to raise awareness and develop a deeper understanding of this invisible disability. Our findings highlight the ignorance about Dyslexia across the education and employment sectors, and society in general, particularly in Australia.

Albert Einstein said:

"I am not more gifted than the average human being. If you know anything about history, you would know that is so--what hard times I had in studying and the fact that I do not have a memory like some other people do... I am just more curious than the average person and I will not give up on a problem until I have found the proper solution. This is one of my greatest satisfactions in life--solving problems--and the harder they are, the more satisfaction do I get out of them. Maybe you could consider me a bit more patient in continuing with my problem than is the average human being. Now, if you understand what I have just told you, you see that it is not a matter of being more gifted but a matter of being more curious and maybe more patient until you solve a problem."

Prologue

This book has been designed for you, the reader, in mind. Each chapter delves into the unique aspects of what life is like for those living with dyslexia and associated neurodivergences, providing in-depth insights and practical advice. To facilitate deeper understanding and engagement, the book includes a series of exercises at the end the chapters. These exercises are crafted to spark meaningful conversations, promote psychological safety and to foster empathy and understanding towards those with neurodivergent conditions.

It is my sincere aspiration that this book will not only serve as an educational resource, but also act as a catalyst for change. By shedding light on the communication barriers and biases that may unintentionally marginalise and devalue individuals with dyslexia and other related conditionsit aims to bring about policy change within the education, health, disability and employment sectors, and a workplace that recognises and supports the unique strengths and challenges of those with dyslexia.

Through these efforts, I hope to foster a more inclusive society where every individual, regardless of their neurodiversity, feels valued and empowered to reach their full potential.

Dyslexia became a passion of mine at the age of 37. At 27,

I was diagnosed with dyslexia and dysgraphia; two labels I did not understand, even though I had trained as a speech pathologist. What became evident as I learnt to live with and understand these labels, was that there was limited formal support for someone like me with this diagnosis. After my diagnosis, I suffered a complete mental breakdown. There was no professional expert or anyone I could talk to; no one I knew, at the time, had dyslexia. I felt dumb, ashamed and I lost my sense of self. I felt that my identity had been stripped from me. I was no longer the person I thought I'd been. After some years of being unwell, with the support of my family, I recovered and started to wonder what happened to all the people like me who didn't recover, that didn't find hope amongst the darkness, who perhaps didn't have the amazing ongoing love and support I had.

Over the years, as I moved from one job to the next, a black cloud of shame followed me; the shame of not being able to read and write like others. As I progressed in my career, I struggled more and more. Because of my dyslexia, I felt I didn't have the writing skills needed for being a manager. Most of my employers appeared to lack the understanding and empathy to help me, and I was frustrated and angry at the systems around me. I felt that three levels of education (primary, secondary and tertiary) had failed me, workplaces were failing me, shaming me, embarrassing me, even questioning my integrity and capacity. There were many nights I cried, feeling lost, unsure of what to do with my life. This uncertainty led me to find clarity, and I was determined to help other people to not feel the isolation, frustration and hurt I had felt throughout my education and employment. This drive led me to undertake my doctorate. I wanted to contribute towards the building of further evidence, desperately needed in Australia, to give a voice to the voiceless and to translate this research into practice. Also, I was hoping to enable Australian society, especially workplaces, to truly see the value of difference, and to be inclusive of all.

I hope this work educates and informs, but most of all, contributes to the start of systemic change across access to the workplace environment, so that those with dyslexia can contribute to society in meaningful ways, and can, as a result, lead healthier, happier and more connected lives.

STANDING ON THE SHOULDERS OF GIANTS

This work acknowledges all those who have gone before me, in particular the dyslexic researchers and our allies. Those who have spent years studying dyslexia in its many shapes and forms, its strengths and difficulties. Those who I've admired from afar and those who I've had the privilege of calling my mentors, friends and guides, with special acknowledgement and thanks to Dr Judith Hudson, Dr Malvika Behl, Dr Neil Alexander-Passe, Dr Helen Ross and Tanya Serry, Lisa Furlong and many other international and local researchers.

Dyslexia research has come a long way from when it was first identified as *word blindness* in the 18th century. Yet, in Australia, there is currently a lack of longitudinal research into the nature of adulthood dyslexia. This means Australia is far behind other developed countries when it comes to understanding their needs. In fact, until now, there has been no research undertaken exploring the lived experiences of Australian adults with dyslexia across the social determinants of health, including healthcare access, educational attainment, employment status, and social and emotional well-being. Further, to my knowledge, there is no Australian research exploring the experiences of employers and managers of dyslexic employees. Through this work, I aim to shed a light on what life is like for Australian adults living with dyslexia and seek to provide recommendations on how their quality-of-life outcomes could be improved.

Being a dyslexic researcher is hard for many reasons: the stigma attached to the belief that dyslexics cannot work in academia, the additional time it takes us to read, put our thoughts coherently on paper and then translate that into research, peer-reviewed papers and more. This is a testament to the sheer grit, perseverance and determination we have to create and contribute to the much-needed research into adulthood dyslexia. My work aims to build on the amazing plethora of research that has been undertaken internationally and is growing in Australia. I am honoured to be contributing to this research and to have been given this remarkable opportunity to Stand on the Shoulders of the dyslexic Giants that have gone before me and to make space for those who come after us because we know there are many.

Background to the research

The adult population with dyslexia represents a considerable portion of the neurodivergent community and 10% of the general populace. Nonetheless, there has been a scarcity of research, conducted in Australia, that examines the experiences of living with this learning disability from the perspective of adults. Research efforts in Australia have primarily been focused on children and adolescents, including topics such as early intervention, educational support, mental health, and well-being. However, as individuals transition into adulthood, a notable gap in research has emerged. Given that dyslexia is recognised as a disability under Australian laws and regulations, it is imperative that research is conducted in Australia to better comprehend how adults with dyslexia navigate their day-to-day lives, and the support they require. Such research provides valuable insights into this cohort and enables the provision of more effective support measures at a policy level.

The objective of my doctoral research was to examine the subjective experiences of adults with dyslexia, with a specific emphasis on their employment status and social and emotional well-being. To achieve this objective, three distinct studies were undertaken. The first study was dedicated to the examination of the social and emotional well-being of adults with dyslexia. The second study was devoted to exploring the workplace experiences of this population. Lastly, the third study sought to investigate the perceptions and experiences of employers and managers, in relation to working with employees who have dyslexia.

The results of the three studies shed light on a range of obstacles encountered by Australian adults with dyslexia. These obstacles, often originating in childhood, persist into adulthood for many individuals, with diagnosis often not occurring until later in life. Despite high levels of education and employment across diverse industries, individuals with dyslexia are subject to substantial disadvantage throughout adulthood, in particular to their employment trajectory, dictating the use of individual coping mechanisms to navigate workplace and daily activities. Because of these pervasive barriers, many individuals experience significant mental health and well-being challenges, lacking opportunities that can enhance their quality of life. This inquiry into dyslexia moves beyond the scope of the traditional medical model. Specifically, in addition to investigating the obvious physiological differences of dyslexia, which predominantly manifest as difficulties in reading, writing and spelling, we aimed to explore its broader ramifications on an individual's self-concept, academic achievements, occupational choices and professional experiences throughout adulthood.

This book yielded additional results from a fourth paper published, investigating the impact of 'labels' on adults with dyslexia through an intersectional lens, as well as other unpublished aspects of this research, such as the social disparity in obtaining a dyslexia diagnosis, the potential of negative educational experiences during childhood leading to traumatic effects, the identification of personal strengths and resources, the role of family support, and the influence of other interpersonal relationships. Intertwined are my own lived experiences of having dyslexia and dysgraphia, as well as my twenty-odd years working as a leader within the health, not-for-profit and social enterprise sectors.

The outcomes derived from this research and lived experiences have been incorporated into a collection of empirical information that can support policymakers, government bodies, and the education, health, and employment sectors in investing in creating more inclusive environments for those with dyslexia and other neurodivergence so they, too, can thrive in our society.

To strengthen this research, we used the application of standardised tools such as the Warwick-Edinburgh Mental Well-being Scales (WEMWBS) [3, 4] and the Job Demands Resource Model of Burnout (JD-R Model) [5, 6]. Globally, the WEMWBS and the JD-R Model have not been used on a sub-population like dyslexia, and this brings a new, exciting, and innovative element to the way we understand the lived experiences of Australian dyslexics and firmly grounds this evidence-based inquiry.

For noting: Throughout the book, there will be quotes from participants and those from the dyslexic community. I will switch between 'person first' dyslexic and 'identify first language' for those with dyslexia. These will be explained further along in the book.

Publications from this research

Wissell, S., Karimi, L. & Serry, T. (2021) Adults with dyslexia: A snapshot of the demands on adulthood in Australia, *Australian Journal of Learning Difficulties*, 26:2, 153-166, DOI: 10.1080/19404158.2021.1991965

Wissell, S., Karimi, L. & Serry, T. Furlong, L & Hudson, H. (2022) "You don't look dyslexic": Using the Job Demands - Resource model to explore workplace experiences of Australian adults with dyslexia. International Journal of Environmental Research and Public Health. S Ed. doi.org/10.3390/ijerph191710719

Wissell, S., Karimi, L. & Serry, T. Furlong, L & Hudson, J. (2022). Leading diverse workforces: Perspectives from managers and employers about dyslexic employees in Australian workplaces. *International Journal of Environmental Research and Public Health. S Ed Dyslexia.* doi.org/10.3390/ijerph191911991

Wissell, S., Hudson, J. Flower, R., & Goh, W (2024) "I hate calling it a disability": Exploring how labels impact adults with dyslexia through an intersectional lens. Under review: *Neurodiversity Journey*

PART ONE
THE JOURNEY INTO
ADULTHOOD

Chapter 1
DYSLEXIA

dyslexia. noun. dys·lex·ia dis-▨lek-sē-▨
a variable often familial learning disability that involves difficulties in
acquiring and processing language and that is typically manifested by a
lack of proficiency in reading, spelling, and writing.
Merriam-Webster Dictionary [7]
Dyslexia (d▨sleksi▨) NOUN
A developmental disorder which can cause learning difficulty in one or
more of the areas of reading, writing, and numeracy.
British English [8]
Dyslexia, (d▨▨leksi▨) NOUN
Pathology: any of various reading disorders associated with impairment
of the ability to interpret spatial relationships or to integrate audito-
ry and visual information.
American English [8]

Dyslexia is a complex condition; it is considered a disability with controversy surrounding it. There are ongoing discussions and debates, both
internally within the dyslexic community, and externally by profes-

sionals, regarding terminology, the validity of dyslexia, the conceptual frameworks we sit within and the appropriate labels to be used. Various labels have been imposed upon us by external entities, including those originating from the medical model, the social model of disability, and the neurodivergent movement. These labels have been applied by the medical and education system, governmental institutions, workplace environments, and through policies and practices, often without our consent. We are currently in a society where our difficulties are not accepted and the environments we are living in are not adaptive to meet our needs; we are therefore disabled in many situations.

Dyslexia is a hidden disability that lacks significant awareness and understanding in education, workplaces and in society. It is a timely reminder of the difficulties many individuals face because of their disabling environment, and how together we can improve these environments, so that everyone can achieve their full potential and live healthier, happier more connected lives. In this chapter, we explore what dyslexia is, how it co-exists with other neurodevelopmental difficulties/differences and the social and emotional challenges linked with dyslexia.

1.1. WHAT IS DYSLEXIA

Originally known as 'word blindness,' dyslexia first came to the attention of the medical fraternity more than 100 years ago when German ophthalmologist, Rudolf Berlin, observed patients having difficulties reading printed words [9, 10]. The difficulty was initially attributed to problems with vision (hence, word blindness), but it was quickly recognised that peripheral visual mechanisms were not the cause, and attention moved to the functions of the brain.

Reading and writing are cultural inventions [11]. They are not innate skills, as is oral language that has been around tens of thousands of years [11]. Reading and writing have only been around for about

4000 - 6000 years [11, 12]. Rather than being born literate, we must learn to read through instruction, deploying parts of our brain that are not naturally suited for that purpose [11, 13].

Figure .1 Dyslexia difficulties

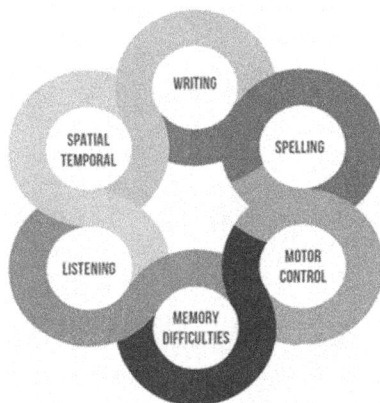

Today, it is understood that dyslexia is a neurobiological condition that affects at least 1 in 10 people in the population [14, 15]. Individuals with dyslexia have a deficit in the mechanism involved in processing phonological information [16-19]. This results in difficulties recognising, identifying and manipulating syllables and phonemes within written language [14, 20, 21], which in turn impacts the ability to recall and decode words accurately and fluently. In addition, dyslexia can affect understanding of orthography (the conventional spelling system of a language), speech perception (e.g., discriminating between sounds such as ba and pa) and the decoding of speech from print [22]. Although primarily impacting reading skills, delays across these different areas of language can lead to secondary effects on spelling and reading comprehension, speed and accuracy, growth of vocabulary and sight vocabulary (words that can be recognised by sight) and background knowledge, as illustrated in Figure 1 [11, 14, 22, 23]. Additionally, numeracy can be impacted as those with dyslexia struggle to understand arithmetic concepts [24]. Recent research conducted by Marks et al. (2024) indicates that deficits in executive functions, particularly variations in visuospatial working memory, are correlated with the presence of concurrent mathematical difficulties. [25].

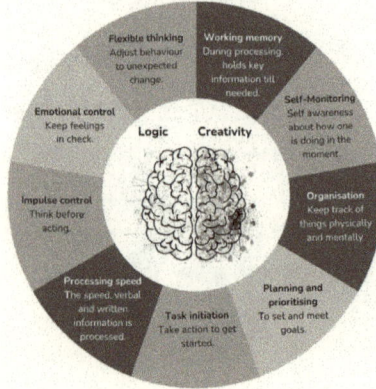

Figure. 2. Executive Functioning and neurodivergence

So, what is executive functioning and how is it linked to dyslexia? Executive function comprises a suite of cognitive abilities encompassing working memory, adaptive thinking, planning and organising, task initiation, problem solving and self-regulation. These skills are instrumental in our everyday activities, facilitating learning, productivity, and the management of daily tasks [26, 27]. A person with dyslexia will have difficulties with different areas of executive function and may show a mixed 'spikey' profile in scores on tests of verbal comprehension, perceptual organisation, working memory and processing speed [9, 28, 29]. These vulnerabilities can lead to challenges in following verbal instructions, maintaining focus, staying organised, adhering to tasks and regulating emotions.

However, it is important to acknowledge that people with dyslexia are not all the same, and variation can occur across the spectrum from mild to severe with external influences impacting day to day functioning, e.g., fatigue, poor mental health, job demands, daily stressors and anxiety [29], (refer to section 2.5). There will be differences depending on the individual, the recentness of their diagnosis, the strength they possess and their coping strategies [29, 30].

What is most important to understand is, that for some people, dyslexia is a crippling disability that will prohibit them from completing school and gaining meaningful employment. They will not learn and work to their intellectual capacity and capability. In today's day and age, where being literate is a basic human right, this is abominable. Research indicates childhood problems associated with reading difficulties, including dyslexia, have consequences on functioning and well-being that persist well into midlife and beyond [31-34]. Furthermore, reading difficulties have been linked to antisocial behaviour and juvenile delinquency, including an over-representation in the justice system [35-39]. The Speech Pathology in Youth (Justice) Custodial Education Project report undertaken at Parkville Youth Corrections Centre in Victoria, Australia found that 40% of incarcerated young people had dyslexia [40]. Globally, we are seeing high rates of dyslexics incarcerated. In 2000, a research study conducted on prisoners in Texas, revealed that 48 percent were diagnosed with dyslexia, and two-thirds faced challenges in reading [41]. These are shocking statistics that need further research to find better ways to reduce the risk of young people disengaging from education and ending up in the justice system.

Dr Neil Alexander-Passee is writing a series of books around neurodivergence and the pipeline into prison - details can be found in the resources section. We need to be doing so much more for those in the justice system when it comes to dyslexia screening and literacy support. So much potential is lost. Why? Why isn't more being done?

How can children progress through their school years and be illiterate in a country like Australia? How are we letting so many children and families down? Why are our governments and policy-makers not specifically addressing this social failing? As you read or listen to the rest of this book, consider the privileged position many of us are in, to attain an education, to be meaningfully employed, and to live a good life. You will come to see the significant disadvantage many dyslexics are facing, as they transition into adulthood, and that so much more should, and must, be done. Understanding these nuances, and the relationship of this disability, highlights that dyslexia encompasses more than solely reading impairments. A comprehensive understanding of this relationship is crucial for the formulation of effective intervention strategies aimed at enabling individuals with dyslexia to reach their full potential.

When I was diagnosed with dyslexia and dysgraphia, I didn't even know what those two words were. Although I was a trained speech pathologist, I hadn't come across the terms. I had learnt about and worked with children who had autism, speech and language disorders, and stuttering. Yet, although dyslexia is such a common difficulty, I hadn't heard of it. *Why?* I wondered. In time, I have become very familiar with these two labels, which still, to this day, cause immense confusion in education, health and workplace settings, even within society as a whole - but we'll get to that later. For now, we know that dyslexia is a noun ... and we can all agree on that, yay!

1.2. CAUSATION

1.2.1. Brain architecture, the neurobiological basis of dyslexia

Figure .3. The Brain architecture for reading. Adapted from Dehaene work.

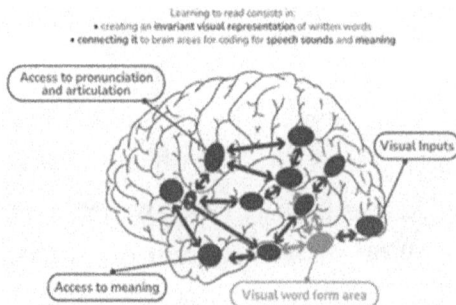

As mentioned earlier, rather than being born literate, we must learn to read and write through instruction, deploying different parts of our brain that are not naturally suited for that purpose [11, 13]. Specifically, the ability to read requires several distinct parts of the left hemisphere of the brain to be active (see Figure .3. adapted from Dehaene [13]) [13, 42]. Evidence indicates that dyslexia is neurologically based. One theory, is that it is caused by under-activity of the left hemisphere's language network, including the occipito-temporal and parieto-temporal areas [11, 43-45]. There are signs of abnormal grey matter and white matter development in the brains of those diagnosed with dyslexia [13, 42]. Magnetic Resonance Imaging (MRI) scans have shown that dyslexics tend to have less grey matter in the left parieto-temporal area, compared to non-dyslexics. A decrease in this area, has been associated with problems with phonological awareness and reduce in reading skills [42]. MRI scans have also indicated that individuals with dyslexia tend to have symmetrical brain structures when compared to the general asymmetrical brains of non-dyslexics [42]. In simple terms, those with dyslexia appear to be born with a different brain structure and composition when compared to the general population.

In recent years, research has established that dyslexia is not caused by poverty, developmental delay, speech, hearing or visual impairments, or learning a second language [42]. Dyslexia is also unrelated to intellectual functioning, with dyslexia occurring across the intellectual quotient (IQ) range of intelligence [46, 47].

1.3. THE INFLUENCE OF GENETICS

There is now considerable evidence that there is a genetic influence involved with dyslexia, and it is often found in more than one member of a family [11, 42, 48-52]. It has also been found that children, who have at least one parent with dyslexia, have a 33% to 66% chance of having dyslexia themselves [49]. Other estimates of familial inheritance range between 50 to 60 percent [51, 53-55]. In my family, we are 100% sure it comes from my dad. One of my siblings has dyslexia, and extended family. Over time, as I have learnt more about autism and ADHD in adults, I can see similar characteristics running through my very neurodiverse and neurodivergent family. Understanding the genetic link is crucial for supporting children, families and adults. Often, parents realise they have dyslexia or neurodivergent traits, only after their child's assessment. Early identification and intervention are essential to improving life outcomes, as reading difficulties are linked to long-term challenges that persist well into midlife and beyond, including poor academic performance, social and emotional issues, and lower occupational status [31, 34, 56-58].

1.4. PREVALENCE

Estimates of the prevalence of dyslexia vary depending on the metrics used for diagnosis. It has been estimated that 7-10% of the global population and some 2.5 million Australians are dyslexic [15, 59-61]. Overseas some counties such as the US and the UK are now saying it is around 20% of the population, or 1 in 5 which is huge [59]! However, in Australia, as the Australian Bureau of Statistics does not collect data on the number of children and adults diagnosed with dyslexia, estimates of prevalence are difficult to confirm. This may change with the advent of the National Consistent Collection of Data (NCCD) introduced and mandated for all schools Australia-wide in 2015, to collect information on students with disabilities, including a learning difficulty, such as dyslexia. Teachers are required to record the number of students within their classroom who have a disability, and what classroom accommodations have been implemented. These recordings are then linked to funding support [62]. Over time this data may provide more accurate information regarding the prevalence of dyslexia in Australia.

1.5. DYSLEXIA AND CO-OCCURRING DIFFICULTIES

As a neurodevelopmental condition, dyslexia may often coexist alongside other developmental disorders, such as speech-sound disorders, language disorders, autism, dyspraxia/developmental coordination disorder (DCD), dyscalculia, dysgraphia, attention deficit hyperactivity disorder (ADHD), and other related conditions encompassed by social and emotional well-being, as illustrated in Figure 4. [48, 54, 63-66]. Comorbidity between developmental disorders in childhood appears to be the norm, rather than the exception [67].

Figure 4. Dyslexia and co-occurring difficulties

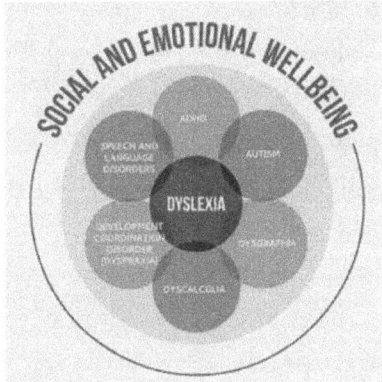

1.5.1. Dyslexia and dyscalculia

Approximately 3–7% of the general population have dyscalculia [68-71]. An individual with dyscalculia can have severe difficulties performing arithmetic calculations that will persist into adulthood, even in the absence of intellectual disability [69, 70]. Dyscalculia leads to marked impairment in academia, work and everyday life, and is linked to co-morbid mental disorders [68, 69]. Between 30-70% of individuals have co-occurring dyslexia and dyscalculia [69, 72]. Although dyslexia and dyscalculia are distinct disorders, working memory weakness, processing speed impairment, and verbal comprehension difficulties are common in both [72].

1.5.2. Dyslexia and dysgraphia

Approximately 3-15% of the general population have dysgraphia; a specific learning condition affecting the written expression of symbols and words [73-75]. Dysgraphia causes motor control difficulties, affecting the motor planning or production processes required for handwriting, visual-spatial difficulties or impairments in acquisition of writing (spelling, handwriting, or both). Dysgraphia can persist despite adequate opportunities to learn, and in the absence of obvious neuropathology or gross sensory–motor dysfunction [73, 74, 76].

People with dysgraphia can have illegible handwriting, difficulty spacing things out on paper or working within margins (poor spatial planning), exhibit frequent erasing and present with inconsistencies in letter and word spacing. They also tend to have poor spelling, including leaving words unfinished or missing words or letters [52, 73, 74, 77]. Although dyslexia and dysgraphia are separate disorders, up to 30% of those with dyslexia will also have dysgraphia [73].

1.5.3. Dyslexia and dyspraxia

Dyspraxia, also known as developmental coordination disorder (DCD), yields difficulties in gross and fine motor coordination and perceptual and spatial-perceptual weaknesses [66]. DCD affects around 5% of the general population and frequently overlaps with other developmental conditions including dyslexia, ADHD and autism [78]. Individuals with DCD commonly have difficulties in several areas, including left-right confusion, tactile perceptual skills, hand-eye coordination, working memory, visual memory, sequencing skills, short-term visual or auditory memory, verbal memory and/or memory for verbal instructions [66]. DCD overlaps with dyslexia and ADHD in 35-50% of cases [79]. While DCD is not commonly associated with difficulty learning to read, it is often associated with significant spelling difficulties [66].

1.5.4. Dyslexia and Autism

Autism is a neurodevelopmental disorder characterised by difficulties with social communication and interaction, as well as restricted, repetitive patterns of behaviour, interests or activities. The severity and presentation of symptoms can vary widely among individuals, and it is estimated to impact about 1% of the general population [80, 81]. Individuals with autism may also exhibit repetitive behaviours. Children and adults with autism are at a higher risk of having co-occurring difficulties such as dyslexia, with the frequency of autism and dyslexia at 20-30% [82].

1.5.5. Dyslexia and Attention-deficit/hyperactivity disorder

Around 5% of the population have Attention-deficit/hyperactivity disorder (ADHD). ADHD, is recognised as three main types: inattention (not being able to keep focus), hyperactivity (excess movement that is not fitting to the setting) and impulsivity (hasty acts that occur in the moment without thought). They can present as one of the following:

- predominantly inattentive
- predominantly hyperactive/impulsive
- a combination of inattention and hyperactive/impulsive

Approximately 25-40% of people with ADHD also have dyslexia [33, 43]. Dyslexia and ADHD often co-occur, meaning that many individuals experience both conditions simultaneously. This co-occurrence can complicate the diagnosis and treatment process, as the symptoms of one condition can overlap or exacerbate the symptoms of the other. Both dyslexia and ADHD are associated with deficits in working memory, which is the ability to hold and manipulate information in the mind over short periods. This can impact reading comprehension, problem-solving and following instructions.

1.5.6. Dyslexia and Developmental Language Disorder

Developmental Language Disorder (DLD), previously known as a specific language impairment (SLI), can co-occur with dyslexia. A multinational and multidisciplinary Delphi consensus study by Bishop and colleagues (2017) established consensus on the preferred terminology for conceptualising language difficulties. Consensus was reached for the use of 'developmental language disorder' (DLD) to describe language difficulties that emerge in the course of development, and are not associated with a known biomedical aetiology and 'language disorder,' used to describe language difficulties that will likely persist beyond childhood and are often associated with known biomedical conditions (e.g., sensorineural hearing loss, Down Syndrome, ASD) [83, 84]. Bishop et al. (2017) noted that dyslexia can co-occur with DLD but that the causal relation is unclear. Therefore, for the purpose of this thesis, DLD will be used. An individual with a DLD has trouble developing structural language, which includes syntax (grammar) and semantics (extracting meaning from words, a phrase or text). DLD and dyslexia are separate neurodevelopmental disorders and the causal relationship is unclear [85]. Individuals with dyslexia and co-occurring DLD have difficulties with oral language, impairments in reading, difficulties with phonological awareness and, generally, they present with more severe difficulties compared to those who only have dyslexia or DLD [86]. The prevalence rates for dyslexia and DLD vary considerably due to age of diagnosis and the criteria used to diagnose these disorders, however rates appear to be between 14-63% [87-89].

DYSLEXIA

1.5.7. Dyslexia and social and emotional well-being

"If we continue to see dyslexia as being merely a reading and writing problem, we will continue to deprive these people of any real understanding or support in terms of the extent and depth of their difficulties."
Laughton King, Author and Educational Child and Family Psychologist

More than half a million Australian children experience significant mental health difficulties annually, with 8.2% of children aged 4-11 diagnosed with a mental health disorder [90, 91]. Half of all mental health disorders emerge before the age of 14, and poor mental health in childhood and adolescence is a predictor of poor mental health in adulthood [92].

A growing body of research, highlights a link between dyslexia and low levels of mental health and well-being [32, 93, 94]. An Australian study by Boyes et al. (2015) suggests that reading difficulties are a risk factor for developing later mental health problems. Children and adolescents with dyslexia face substantial psychosocial and emotional challenges throughout their schooling years, including feelings of stigma, discrimination, alienation, shame and isolation [94-96].

Early experiences of struggle and continued failure in foundational academic areas, such as reading and writing, may have damaging life-long effects [97]. Dyslexia is independently associated with lower levels of well-being [98] and higher rates of anxiety, depression and suicidal ideation, even when controlling for other disorders such as ADHD [99, 100]. Individuals with dyslexia are twice as likely to experience anxiety and depression [101, 102] and are 47% more likely to attempt suicide compared to the general population [103, 104].

The significant mental health challenges faced by those with dyslexia, underscore the urgent need for early intervention and support. The

World Health Organization estimates that untreated mental health conditions contribute to 13% of the total global burden of disease. It is anticipated that by 2030, mental health issues, particularly depression, will become the leading cause of mortality and morbidity worldwide [105]. The link between dyslexia and adverse mental health outcomes that start in childhood, highlights the profound impact of early academic struggles on long-term well-being. Children with dyslexia not only contend with the academic difficulties associated with reading and writing but also face substantial psychosocial and emotional challenges, including stigma, discrimination and isolation.

This growing body of research makes it clear that dyslexia is not merely an academic issue, but a significant public health concern that demands comprehensive and sustained support strategies. Addressing these challenges requires a multifaceted approach that includes early identification, effective educational interventions, and robust mental health support systems. By acknowledging and addressing the complex interplay between dyslexia and mental health, we can better support children, young people and adults in overcoming their difficulties and achieving their full potential. Further exploration of mental health and well-being, in relation to dyslexia, will be discussed in Chapters three and seven.

1.6. CONCLUSIONS

Dyslexia is a complex, neurobiological condition that is much broader than just reading difficulties, affecting at least 1 in 10 individuals. Dyslexia is linked to structural and functional abnormalities in the brain, particularly within the left hemisphere's language network. Often genetic in nature, dyslexia is marked by challenges in phonological processing, which impairs the ability to decode and recall words, impacting reading fluency, speed and comprehension, and can also affect other areas such as orthography, speech perception and numeracy skills.

Despite these challenges, it is crucial to recognise the variability in dyslexia's presentation, influenced by factors such as severity, individual strengths, coping strategies, and external conditions, like mental health and daily stressors. Dyslexia is linked to co-occurring neurodevelopmental conditions, including ADHD, autism, and other learning disabilities, each bringing its own set of challenges that can compound the difficulties faced by those with dyslexia. Recognising dyslexia's wide-ranging impact across executive functions, from working memory to emotional regulation, is necessary for developing effective interventions, workplace support and understanding. Recognising the profound impact of dyslexia on mental health and overall well-being is also vital. These interventions must be tailored to address both the academic, workplace performance and socio-emotional aspects of dyslexia, aiming to support individuals in achieving their full potential.

The terminology and diagnostic criteria for dyslexia continue to change over time, reflecting growing awareness and understanding of the condition. Nevertheless, these changes have created vagueness in education, health, employment, and society as a whole. This highlights the need for a consistent and clear definition of dyslexia to ensure appropriate support and accommodations. By addressing these multifaceted challenges, we can foster environments where individuals with dyslexia can thrive academically, socially, and emotionally.

KEY TAKE-HOME MESSAGES

Historical Evolution: Previously known as "word blindness," dyslexia has moved from being associated with problems with vision to being acknowledged as a neurological disorder that affects 1 in 10 Australians.

Cultural Invention of Reading and Writing: The acquisition of reading and writing skills is a comparatively recent development in human history, necessitating the use of brain functions that are not naturally appropriate for these tasks.

Impact on Language Skills: Dyslexia significantly impacts language skills, including phonological processing, orthography and decoding, ultimately influencing reading, spelling and comprehension.

Diverse Profile and External Factors: The chapter acknowledges the diverse profile of individuals with dyslexia, influenced by external factors, and recognises a spectrum of severity.

Terminology and Classification Challenges: The evolving terminology, diagnostic criteria and classification of dyslexia as a disability, present both benefits and challenges, particularly in the Australian context.

Importance of Inclusive Environments: Recognition of dyslexia as part of neurodiversity underscores the need for inclusive environments and support systems.

Global Prevalence Challenges in Australia: The chapter explores the prevalence of dyslexia globally, emphasising challenges in obtaining accurate data, particularly in the Australian context due to challenges with the types of labels used about dyslexia.

Co-occurrence with Neurodevelopmental Conditions: Dyslexia is associated with other neurodevelopmental conditons, including dyscalculia, dysgraphia, dyspraxia, ADHD, autism and developmental language disorder.

Increased Understanding: The chapter provides a comprehensive overview, aiming to increase one's understanding of dyslexia and the complexity it brings to different areas of life.

Connection with Mental Health: Dyslexia is strongly interconnected with mental health and well-being, urging a shift from viewing it merely as a reading and writing problem.

Urgency in Addressing Psychosocial Challenges: The chapter emphasises the urgency of addressing psychosocial challenges faced by individuals with dyslexia, setting the stage for further exploration into the intricate relationship between dyslexia and mental health in subsequent sections.

Complexities and Profound Impact: A deeper understanding of dyslexia's complexities and its profound impact on various aspects of human experience emerges, laying the groundwork for a nuanced exploration in subsequent chapters.

RESOURCES

There are a huge number of resources you can find so we are listing just a few to help you on your journey of discovery and understanding. You can find more information at re:think dyslexia.com.au. If you found any of this content distressing, please seek support:

- Lifeline Australia - 13 11 14
- Beyond Blue - 1300 22 4636
- NEAP Neurodivergent Employment Assistance Program - 1800 13 6327

Organisations supporting neurodivergent adults:

- **re:think dyslexia**
- ADHD Australia
- Neurodiversity Hub
- Untapped Holding

Books, podcasts and more
Dr Judith Hudson,

- A Practical Guide to Congenital Developmental Disorders and Learning Difficulties

Dr Neil Alexander-Passe books:

- ADHD and Crime: Investigating the 'School to Prison Pipeline' (Dio Press) –
- Dyslexia, Neurodiversity, and Crime: Investigating the 'School to Prison Pipeline' (Dio Press)
- Surviving school as a dyslexic teenager: A guide for parents
- **Dear Dyslexic Podcast** on your favoured podcast platform and subscribe, rate, and review.

Relevant Dear Dyslexic podcast episodes:
- Episode 69 Melissa Webster "From Diagnosis to CEO: Mel Webster's Journey with ADHD and Dyslexia.
- Episode 28 out now with American Actor, Author and Dyslexia Advocate Ameer Baraka

Chapter 2
DYSLEXIA, LABELS AND MODELS

I don't have a dis-ability, I have a different-ability
- Robert M. Hensel

This chapter examines how labels and theoretical frameworks provide insights into the experiences of dyslexic adults. Different societal perspectives on dyslexia influence identity and self-determination. The medical model, highlighted by the DSM-5, utilises diagnostic labels for categorisation, aiding in diagnosis, treatment and health data collection, while also offering validation to individuals and families, particularly in late diagnoses.

However, these diagnostic labels can perpetuate stigma and misconceptions about dyslexia. Historical understandings of dyslexia, shaped by biological, psychological and social factors, complicate label use, often overshadowing broader psychological and social elements. Frameworks, like the social model of disability, analyse the psychosocial impacts of dyslexia, while Bronfenbrenner's Ecological

Model addresses the complexities of human experiences in varied environments.

Intersectionality theories further enrich the understanding of dyslexic adults by considering gender, ethnicity and socioeconomic status. By integrating these perspectives, we gain a comprehensive view of dyslexia in adulthood, informing tailored interventions and support systems. This chapter explores the evolution of labels from medical diagnostics to cultural concepts like neurodiversity, examining their implications for dyslexic individuals in the workplace, including issues of disclosure, accommodation and stigma.

2.1. MEDICAL MODEL

Dyslexia and its co-occurring difficulties are traditionally derived from the medical model of health; a model that has dominated how society conceptualises health and well-being since the 18th century [106]. The medical model views health as an attribute measured by whether disease is present or not; that is, the absence of disease equals good health.

Under the medical model, dyslexia has been classified using a variety of labels, including a specific reading disability, specific reading disorder, specific learning impairment, learning disability or specific learning disorder/difficulty [14, 43, 107-114]. The Diagnostic and Statistical Manual Fifth Edition (DSM-5) – the reference handbook for mental disorders – provides the following distinction:

*"Specific learning disorder, often referred to as 'learning disorder' is a medical term used for diagnosis. 'Learning disability' is a term used by both the educational and legal systems. Though learning disability is not exactly synonymous with specific learning disorder, someone with a diagnosis of specific learning disorder can expect to meet criteria for a learning disability and have the legal status of a federally recognized disability to qualify for accommodations and services in school" [115].*In Australia,

'learning difficulties' and 'learning disabilities' are the accepted – if inconsistent – terms used to describe dyslexia across the education and higher education sectors, and amongst health professionals including general practitioners, educational, clinical psychologists and speech pathologists. Specific reading disability or specific reading disorder is by far the most common type of learning disability, accounting for approximately 80% of all learning disabilities [15]. These terms are often used interchangeably to describe this reading deficit; however, they have caused confusion within the medical and education professionals and the wider public. Under the Discrimination Act, the term 'specific learning disability' is the umbrella term used to describe dyslexia, dyscalculia and dysgraphia [111, 116]. However, terms used are different between states and territories in Australia. For example, in New South Wales, the term learning difficulty is legislated under the Educational Support for Children with Significant Learning Difficulties Bill 2008 [111]. While in Victoria, the State Government uses the term specific learning difficulties to encompass dyslexia, dysgraphia, dyscalculia, developmental coordination disorder and ADHD [117].

The DSM-5 outlines three types of learning disorders: deficits in reading, deficits in writing and deficits in mathematics [118]. While the DSM-5 attempted to streamline terminology and diagnosis, the definitions still leave themselves open to ambiguity. The International Classification of Diseases provides similar criteria for diagnosing dyslexia but also includes underdeveloped reading comprehension skills [119]. Given that dyslexia is classified as a "disability", individuals with this diagnosis are protected under Australian disability-related legislation, including the Disability Discrimination Act 1992, Fair Work Act 2010 and the Equal Opportunity Act 2010 [116, 120, 121]. While this protection brings with it many benefits, the labelling of dyslexia as a disability is not universally accepted [122, 123], and brings with it other considerations (see 3.6.1.1 *Labels and their impact*). Under the medical model paradigm, the focus of dyslexia's impact is on the physiological. This includes issues with reading and writing, verbal comprehension, perceptual organisation, working memory, processing speed, motor control, and concentration [9, 28, 29].

However, it is important to acknowledge that people with dyslexia are not all the same, and variation can occur across the spectrum (i.e., people may experience mild to severe difficulties that cause varying degrees of functional impact) [29].

2.2. SOCIAL MODEL OF DISABILITY

The social model of disability was created to object to the concept of the medical model, which states that a disability is a medical condition that needs to be "fixed" [124-126]. As an alternative, the Social Model of Disability argues that "people with impairments are disabled/excluded by a society that is not organised in ways that take account of their needs" [127]. That is, disabilities result from physical and social barriers in society that limit or take away opportunities for people to participate on an equal basis with others [128].

Over the last thirty years, the social model has been successful in political activism, but it has not been free of criticism [124, 126], some of which has come from within the disability community. It has been argued that the model focuses too much on physical impairment and excludes those with learning difficulties or other adjustment disorders that may appear as 'invisible' disability [124, 129].

In more recent years, as the association between dyslexia and mental health and well-being has become more apparent, there has been growing recognition that the impact of dyslexia is far broader and more complex than the original focus on learning deficits. This understanding of dyslexia's impact on mental health has coincided with a greater understanding of how people's sociological context (the social, cultural and political environments in which people live) affect how they live. For people with dyslexia, 'societal barriers' such as prejudice, stigma, a lack of awareness or understanding, and social exclusion can all affect how dyslexia will impact a person throughout their life [130-134]. The multi-dimensional nature of the impact of dyslexia is now being explored in various models of disability [28, 133].

2.3. NEURODIVERGENCE IS MORE THAN AUTISM AND ADHD

A small amount of literature has discussed dyslexia within a sociological framework [129, 133, 135-138]. Dyslexia has been positioned within this framework to raise the profile of dyslexia and to try and reduce discrimination, stigma and marginalisation by breaking down barriers and transforming societal attitudes. [124, 139]. Recently, we have witnessed the emergence of the term and concept of "neurodiversity", a *non-medical* term coined by Judy Singer in the late 1990s [140, 141]. Initially, thesis research undertaken by Singer looked to draw on her lived experience of three generations of autistic women within her family. Looking beyond the autistic difficulties to the many strengths of autistic individuals. The term neurodiversity has evolved into a symbolic representation of a significant social movement in the 21st century [142]. While Singer did not provide a specific definition for neurodiversity, others have expanded the term, often in alignment with the Social Model of Disability. According to Walker (2023), advocates of the neurodiversity paradigm refrain from using pathologising terms such as 'disorder' to describe neurocognitive differences like autism and

ADHD [140]. This paradigm, then, serves as a positive affirmation of difference, challenging the notion that variations are inherently dysfunctional [30, 143, 144].

We have moved beyond the term neurodiversity to 'neurodivergence' as everyone is neurodiverse. Just like the ecosystem is diverse in nature, so are human beings. However, those with dyslexia, ADHD and autism have diverged from the diverse. As framed by Walker (2023), neurodivergence is not a trait but rather a state where an individual or group diverges from the dominant societal neurocognitive functioning to encompass various neurodevelopmental and co-occurring difficulties such as dyslexia, dysgraphia, dyscalculia, developmental coordination disorder/dyspraxia, ADHD, Tourette's syndrome [140]. Notably, the term is now expanding to include mental health conditions like bipolar disorder and chronic post-traumatic stress syndrome, introducing a layer of complexity. However, when in the workplace, the term and concept is heavily slanted towards those with Autism, and now ADHD, and those with learning difficulties like dyslexia are left out in the cold. Why I wonder? Why are dyslexics not getting a seat at the neurodivergent table?

Yet moving beyond the social model of disability, the concept of neurodiversity as a label does not resonate with all dyslexics. This is despite the growing focus of the global neurodivergence movement, the concept now being embedded within educational, health and employment programs, and increasing media and social media attention. The use of a neurodiversity label can overlook the individual disability of dyslexia when applying a non-medical umbrella term. Neurodevelopment conditions, mental health conditions and chromosomal disorders, such as Down Syndrome and intellectual disabilities, have now all been placed under the umbrella term of neurodivergence. This waters down the strengths and lifelong difficulties faced by those with these conditions/differences and can create societal expectations within education and the workplace with a one-size-fits-all approach. There are significant differences in abilities between someone with Down Syndrome and someone with dyslexia, and we are now seeing a power struggle play out on platforms such as LinkedIn and Facebook, where the loudest neurodivergent voices who don't represent dyslexics are being heard.

My research found that those with dyslexia did not associate with the term neurodiversity or neurodivergence [145]. This could leave many in the dyslexic community feeling disconnected from the narrative within the neurodivergent cultural movement as well as the medical and Social Model of Disability. This disconnection leaves those within the dyslexic community feeling that their needs and experiences are not being heard or fully represented. I sometime feel that the loudest voices with the most power, such as those advocating for neurodivergent identities or those in authoritative positions. This research highlights the need to explore the impact of labels and cultural movements that dyslexics get caught up in. This is a fraught issue, best left for debate on another day.

The *Bronfenbrenner Ecological Model* and Intersectionality are two theoretical frameworks that can be applied to better understand the complexities of dyslexia and how different aspects of one's life, including education, employment attainment, government policy, family dynamics and socioeconomic status can all play a part in our quality-of-life outcomes. These frameworks are both used across academia and policy to explain complex issues in society. This short chapter provides an overview of how these two models can be applied to gain a greater and more deeper understanding of dyslexia and how we can talk about dyslexia at a systems and processes level and within policy.

2.4. BRONFENBRENNER ECOLOGICAL MODEL

Figure 5. Bronfenbrenner Ecological Model, 1974

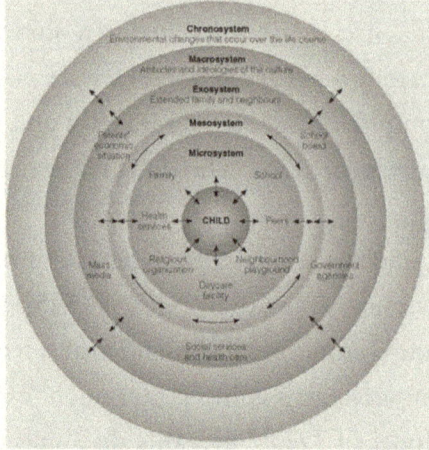

The ecological model is defined by five concentric circles or systems: the *microsystem*; *mesosystem; exosystem, macrosystem* and *chronosystem* [146]. The original model depicts how each system either influences or is influenced by the next (and sometimes both) (see Figure 5). Ecological systems theory and the ecological model address some of the key failings of the medical and social models through their depiction of the complexities of human life within an ever-evolving social, cultural and political environment. This has implications for numerous groups within society, including people with dyslexia [146, 147]. This adapted model places the dyslexic at the centre of circular layers of influence, which represent the various circumstances that can impact dyslexic adults (Figure 6). Adopting Bronfenbrenner's ecological model is a useful tool in providing a more nuanced understanding of the interplaying factors that contribute to the lived experiences of dyslexia. When looking at it from a dyslexic perspective, Bronfenbrenner's model highlights the importance of considering these interrelating levels of influence that can impact a dyslexic, including how they feel about themselves and what they internalise and externalise, the direct environment around them (such as family, peers and work), and broad-er societal and cultural factors [147, 148]. Each of these systems will be explored separately in more detail. The Bronfenbrenner Ecological Model enriches our comprehension by depicting the complexities of human life within social, cultural and political environments. Placing individuals with dyslexia at the core, this adapted model recognises the diverse factors that can influence their lives. By acknowledging the multi-dimensional nature of dyslexia, the ecological model can be used to address some of the shortcomings of medical and social models by emphasising how the interplay of various influences at different levels impacts a dyslexic's life. This is a new way of thinking about the impact of dyslexia which hasn't been done well to date.

2.5. INTERSECTIONALITY

Kimberlé Crenshaw created the Intersectional Framework, which highlighted the marginalisation of black women in antidiscrimination law, feminist theory and anti-racist movements in the United States [149]. This framework emphasises the need to recognise the unique challenges faced by marginalised and disadvantaged communities and individuals [149]. Intersectionality examines how different character-istics of one's identity crisscross, shaping experiences of privilege and oppression. It can used to frame the different experiences that those with dyslexia face in how they view their lives as either a life of privilege or oppression, which has never been done before.

Utilising the Intersectionality Framework within the dyslexic pop-ulation showcases and enables a broader understanding of the com-plicated nature of dyslexic identity and explains how the interplay of diverse social categories contributes to individuals' complex experienc-es of privilege and oppression [145]. This theoretical tool encourages critical thinking that moves beyond the diagnostic categorisation of dyslexia as merely a reading disorder, instead highlighting the interactions of identity factors such as race, gender, class, sexual orientation and ability, as well as the implications of power and privilege in facilitating success for some individuals, while others contend with the challenges associated with dyslexia. Let's look at an example of three different people who all have dyslexia.

Female one: Caucasian woman with dyslexia and dysgraphia, diagnosed in early adulthood. Finished university degree but is under-employed as a disability worker as she can't pass the psychometric testing to work as a nurse. She has a partner with three children, two of whom are neurodivergent. She won't share her difficulties with her workplace due to fear of losing her job. She is struggling with her mental health but can't afford to access support.

Female two: Middle eastern woman who wasn't diagnosed until her 40s. She completed year 10 and English is her second language. She can only work part-time because she is a single mum. She won't share her difficulties with her workplace and friends because its culturally shameful to not be able to read and write. She feels isolated and stupid, although now she knows why she has struggled all her life.

Male one: Caucasian male, diagnosed in primary school and had access to early intervention. Went on to university, now works in an executive role. Has shared his disability with his EA and team, where he accesses workplace accommodations and sees his dyslexia as a strength that he can draw from to undertake his job role.

All three have dyslexia, but examining these examples through an intersectional lens, reveals how experiences of privilege and oppression uniquely shape everyone's identity and life circumstances.

Female one could be viewed as at a disadvantage because she is female, however, in a more privileged position because she is Caucasian. She was diagnosed with dyslexia and dysgraphia in early adulthood, so this could have an impact on her mental health and well-being, her sense of self and coming to terms with the disability label. It also exemplifies how systemic barriers in professional environments, such as psychometric testing, can lead to under-employment. Despite her educational achievements, she remains in a job below her qualifications, fears job loss if she discloses her difficulties, and struggles with mental health issues without access to support and the baggage of a diagnosis in early adulthood.

Female two, could be viewed as already being at a disadvantage because she is a female from a culturally linguistically-diverse background. She has had a late diagnosis, in her 40s, which can have significant impacts on her ability to attain an education and gain meaningful employment. This impacts on social and emotional well-being. This also highlights how cultural stigmas around literacy and neurodivergence can exacerbate feelings of isolation and inadequacy. Her limited educational attainment and the demands of being a single mother, restrict her to part-time work, and cultural shame prevents her from seeking understanding or support in her community and workplace.

In contrast, male one, could be seen as already in a privileged position because he is a Caucasian male. Being diagnosed in primary school, he has benefited from an early diagnosis and intervention. He has built the self-awareness and advocacy skills needed to get through life with an understanding of what tools and strategies will support him. He now thrives in an executive role and is financially secure. We see more males in executive roles than female, although the gender gap is becoming smaller. His ability to disclose his dyslexia and receive workplace accommodations illustrates how support and acceptance can transform dyslexia into a perceived strength and source of resilience.

These examples highlight the critical importance of recognising and addressing the intersecting factors of race, gender, socio-economic status and cultural background in understanding the varied impacts of dyslexia, as seen in my research [145]. Such an intersectional approach is essential for developing comprehensive support systems that acknowledge and mitigate these diverse challenges. Although intersectionality has been applied within other disability communities, such as those with autism [150-152], its application within the dyslexic community remains under-explored, until now [145], and should be acknowledged as a framework for policymakers, education and employment sectors. This concept is further examined in Chapter 3.2.2, which focuses on the implications of labelling.

2.6. CONCLUSION

This chapter walks you through the different theoretical frameworks that can be applied to gain a better understanding of the complexities of adulthood dyslexia. Together, we explored the ever-changing terminology in the medical model and the move towards the Social Model of Disability and the move toward the all-encompassing language around neurodivergence and the implications this can have in watering down the difficulties faced by those placed under this umbrella term. By looking at dyslexia through different frameworks we move beyond it being just a learning disability that only impacts reading. It enables a richer understanding of the context for examining the impact of dyslexia within the broader social frameworks. It also illustrates the challenges of the varying models and frameworks used to explain dyslexia and how this can create confuse, not just within the dyslexic community, but for those across education, health, employment and society.

I don't blame you if you feel somewhat overwhelmed and exhausted after this chapter because there is so much to take in, and you can see how the changing terminology and theories can cause angst and confusion within the dyslexic community and beyond. If anything, the key take-home can be helpful in summarising what you have just learnt and can be shared with those around you. The Dear Dyslexic Podcasts with Dr Love will also help you unpack *intersectionality* more as well!

KEY TAKE-HOME MESSAGES

Understanding of Dyslexia: The chapter emphasises the need for a nuanced understanding of dyslexia, considering its multifaceted nature, influenced by biological, psychological and social factors.

Drawbacks of Labels: While labels are crucial for diagnosis and communication, they may carry societal stigmas and oversimplify the complexities of dyslexia, influencing how it is comprehended and addressed.

Social Model's Contribution: The social model of disability broadens the focus beyond physiological impacts, highlighting societal barriers and psychosocial aspects that shape the experiences of individuals with dyslexia.

Neurodiversity Paradigm: The neurodiversity paradigm challenges pathologising terms, celebrating the positive aspects of neurocognitive variations, but the shift toward 'neurodivergence' introduces complexity, potentially leaving certain conditions, like dyslexia, marginalised.

Ecological Model's Holistic Perspective: The Bronfenbrenner Ecological Model offers a holistic perspective, considering various factors influencing the lives of individuals with dyslexia at different levels within their environment.

Intersectionality Matters: The intersectionality framework underscores the importance of considering the nuanced interactions of various aspects of a dyslexic's identity, contributing to a more inclusive perspective on the experiences of individuals with dyslexia.

In essence, the chapter advocates for a comprehensive and empathetic approach to understanding dyslexia, considering the interplay of biological, psychological and social factors, and highlighting the importance of inclusive frameworks for individuals with dyslexia in various aspects of life.

Chapter 3

THE DYSLEXIC JOURNEY TO THE WORKPLACE THROUGH THE LENS OF BRONFENBRENNER

"I've learned that people will forget what you said, people will forget what you did, but people will never forget how you made them feel."

Maya Angelou

Figure 6. Adaptation of the Bronfenbrenner Ecological Systems Model, for use with dyslexic adult populations (2023)

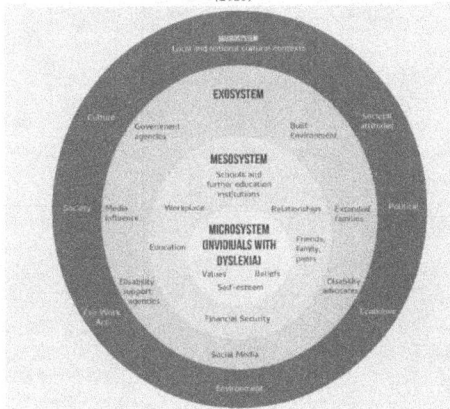

This chapter is huge and has been broken up into sections to help you explore the different touch points throughout a person's life and their journey into adulthood, discovering the key aspects that link across the *microsystem; mesosystem; exosystem, and macrosystem* of Bronfenbrenner's model and *Intersectionality* within these systems. At the *macrosystem,* we address the societal influences that shape the way we view dyslexia. At the exosystem, we look at access to services and diagnosis, as well as the role early diagnosis and intervention has on quality of life outcomes, funding inequality, access to services and early intervention, and the factors that influence us as we transition into the workplace as a young adult. The mesosystem, reports on the negative impact of the education system, the importance of family and being connected with peers and those around us. And then, at the core - the microsystem - we look at how society influences and shapes the way we think and feel about ourselves. This chapter lays the foundations for the following sections on dyslexia in the workplace.

3.1. THE MACROSYSTEM

Figure 8. Dyslexia across the lifespan from my research.

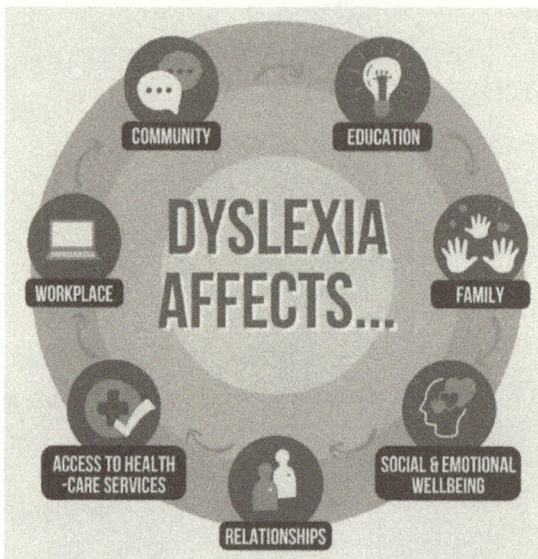

The macrosystem (outermost circle) encompasses the broader societal-level influences on individuals' lives. These include our cultures, societal attitudes and laws, political ideologies, economic factors, technological advancements, and the environment [153]. In Bronfenbrenner's model of child development, it is the microsystem (family, school, neighbourhood) that is considered most influential, with the macrosystem influencing the child more indirectly [153]. However, in adulthood the macrosystem exerts a more direct influence on an individual. An example of the macrosystem is the way society views and treats difference and disability, with society often following its lead from the political ideology of the government of the day - this being a particularly important aspect of the macrosystem. Societal attitudes toward dyslexia can contribute to stigma and misconceptions. Lack of awareness and understanding may lead to negative stereotypes, potentially affecting how individuals with dyslexia are perceived and treated by others. Figure 8 highlights how dyslexia affects and intersects across the social determinants and the ecological model.

Section 3.1 and 3.2.2 will look at different political, legal and societal influences, that can impact the way those with dyslexia can live their lives to their full potential. Now some of this may be a bit controversial, but if we don't critically think about these issues, we will never progress our thinking of adulthood dyslexia.

3.1.1. Political systems

Socio-economic status plays a role in one's ability to access an assessment and early interventions. Local research demonstrates that over 58% of people are not being diagnosed until adulthood in Australia [98], while in the U.K research by Ross highlighted that 80% of young people were not diagnosed until after they left school. There is an apparent inequality between neurodevelopmental conditions in relation to funding and support. Although dyslexic people make up 50% of the neurodivergent population, they receive the least amount of access to funding and support, compared to other neurodevelopmental conditions such as autism, which is covered under the the National Disability Insurance Scheme (NDIS) and the Australian Medicare Benefits Scheme (MBS).

In Australia, the cost of a diagnostic assessment for dyslexia is upward of A$1,500 [154]. Following diagnosis, access to private health professionals such as speech pathologists and educational support, such as private tutors, can be anywhere from $60.00-$200.00 per session. These costs may be unaffordable as dyslexia and learning disabilities are not covered under the NDIS nor the MBS. The failure of the Australian Government to provide appropriate resources has resulted in an expectation, and a heavy reliance on parents or the dyslexic person themself, to be able to advocate and pay for a diagnosis and, then, any interventions that may be needed [155]. This incongruent treatment of different disabilities contributes to social injustice via economic inequity. Figure 9 illustrates the concept between equity and equality. The concept of equality suggests that every individual or group is provided with the same resources or opportunities, while equity acknowledges that each person has unique circumstances and distributes resources and opportunities according to their specific needs to achieve an equal outcome. This research identifies that individuals with dyslexia encounter significant social inequities due to their lack of access to essential resources and opportunities needed to accommodate their disabilities. Consequently, numerous children fail to receive adequate support, and as they transition into adulthood, they experience difficulties in reading, writing and mathematics. This can result in enduring consequences for their educational attainment, employment prospects, mental health and overall quality of life. It is imperative that further action is taken.

As you read or listen to the subsequent chapters, you will witness the daily struggles faced by adults with dyslexia, along with their strength, resilience and perseverance in constructing fulfilling lives with minimal support. The question you should ask yourself as you work your way through this book is *Why?* Why are there such systemic barriers being placed in front of dyslexic children, young people and adults, compared to other conditions?

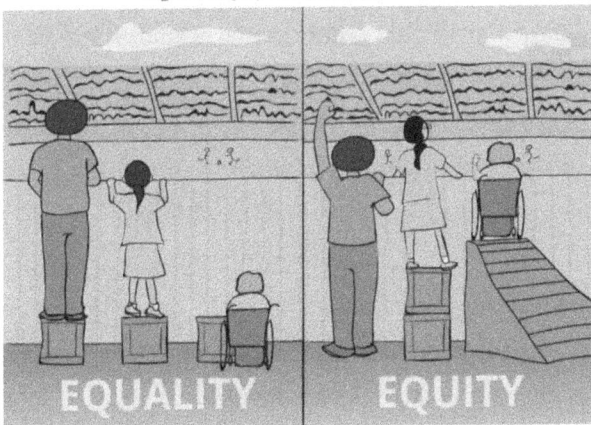

Figure 9. Equity vs. Equality [2]

$63,000
Is the maximum penalty for each act of unlawful discrimination for a workplace.
Fair Work, 2017

3.1.2. Legal influences

Learning disabilities, like dyslexia, can be recognised as 'disabilities' under the *Disability Discrimination Act 1992* (Cth) (**DDA**). Where they are, then the DDA prohibits less favourable treatment in certain areas of life, including employment, education and provision of goods and services. There are also provisions in the *Fair Work Act 2009* (Cth) that prohibit and penalise disability discrimination by employers.

There are four main types of behaviour that the DDA prohibits:

1. Direct discrimination - treating a person with disability less favorably because of their disability. It can also include a failure to make a reasonable adjustment for a person with disability.
2. Indirect discrimination – imposing a requirement or condition (even inadvertently) where the effect is a person with disability cannot comply with that requirement or condition and it was not reasonable in the circumstances to impose the requirement or condition. Like direct discrimination, it can also include a failure to make a reasonable adjustment for a person with disability.
3. Harassment – where a person with disability experiences repeated acts of direct and/or indirect discrimination.
4. Victimisation – where a person who has brought a discrimination complaint or has told their employer they are proposing to, is treated less favourably or adversely because of that.

There are exemptions in the DDA that employers can rely on to justify or excuse direct and indirect discrimination. The main three, in the employment context, are:

1. where the employer can prove that the conduct is reasonable in all the circumstances of the case
2. where the employer can prove that to prevent the discrimination would have caused it unjustifiable hardship
3. where the employer can prove that the employee with disability cannot perform the inherent requirements of the role for which they are employed.

The Fair Work Act also provides an avenue for employees with disability to pursue formal legal proceedings where they have been subjected to unlawful discrimination. Those provisions are referred to as 'General Protections' in the Act. An employee with disability who has been subjected to unlawful discrimination may have rights to pursue formal proceedings in the Fair Work Commission or the Court under the Act. If a person considers they have been unlawfully discriminated against at work by their employer, they should seek prompt legal advice.

Dyslexia discrimination and workplace law

Education and awareness around disability and workplace adjustments is an important way to reduce workplace discrimination. Regrettably, workplaces often lack awareness and understanding about dyslexia, and the adjustments needed for employees with dyslexia. This can have work health and safety consequences. Employers need to listen to staff with dyslexia and be more proactive to identify support and adjustments for employees. The goal ought to be inclusive practice across the employment life cycle.

Whole of organisation disability awareness training can assist employers and their staff to meet obligations under the DDA and other laws. Psychologically safe work environments need to be provided that ideally include awareness raising, mental health support, understanding and access to reasonable adjustments across the employment life cycle. This in turn will reduce job burnout and provide a return on investment with higher productivity levels, whilst also creating greater job satisfaction for all staff.

Since the turn of the century, there has been a cultural shift globally and nationally regarding the need to increase community awareness and greater inclusion of people with disabilities. Both disability and inclusion are paramount underpinnings of the United Nations Convention on the Rights of Persons with Disability (UNCRPD), to which Australia is a signatory. As such, the Australian Government has a responsibility to promote policy that protects the human rights and inherent dignity of people with disability. Australia's commitment to this is confirmed by it being a signatory. Article 27 of the UNCRPD, "Work and employment", recognises:

'the right of persons with disabilities to work, on an equal basis with others; this includes the right to the opportunity to gain a living by work freely chosen or accepted in a labour market and work environment that is open, inclusive and accessible to persons with disabilities'

In Australia, the establishment of the National Disability Insurance Scheme (NDIS) and the National Disability Strategy 2021–2031 [156] has progressed a broader national conversation about how we value and support people with disability. Australian legislation has also helped to drive cultural change, most notably the DDA and parts of the Fair Work Act.

However, there is still progress to be made. For example, under the NDIS, learning disabilities, such as dyslexia, generally are not recognised or considered as a basis for funding. There is also no collection of data on the number of people diagnosed with dyslexia beyond the age of 16 (up to age 16, data is collected through the National Consistent Collection of Data or NCCD described elsewhere - see Chapter 3.3 *Prevalence* of this thesis, p.36). Without data, it is difficult to guide national disability policies and strategies. While legislation is important, enforcement of legislation and other regulations is equally important if the rights of people with disability are to be upheld, including those with dyslexia. This could also reduce stigmatisation, particularly if awareness about dyslexia is raised in the community [100, 139, 157-164].

The lack of recognition of dyslexia under Australia's NDIS, yet recognition in other contexts, such as disability discrimination law, creates confusion and adversely impacts societal understanding of dyslexia and how it affects those who live with it. Improving community attitudes is critical for those with all types of disabilities, including dyslexia, to feel accepted and valued as members of society [165, 166]. However, despite dyslexia being one of the most prevalent disabilities in Australia, there remains a significant lack of awareness and understanding of it across many sectors, particularly the employment sector.

Our aim, is to have high levels of awareness in organisations that lead to responsive support systems in place, as well as high psychological safety. When individuals feel high levels of psychological safety, we know that they can perform at their best. When we have little to low awareness of dyslexia and how to support employees, we usually see little to no systems in place, leading to job burnout as discussed earlier.

CASE STUDIES
At the end of this chapter there are two case studies (pseudonyms used) which highlight discrimination in the workplace, taken from my research and work with dyslexic individuals.

CONCLUSION
This section explores the journey of individuals with dyslexia through the lens of Bronfenbrenner's ecological systems theory, covering the microsystem, mesosystem, exosystem, and macrosystem, while also considering intersectionality within these systems. The chapter highlights the key aspects of how societal, political and legal factors shape the lives of individuals with dyslexia, particularly as they transition into adulthood.

In the macrosystem, societal attitudes toward dyslexia contribute to stigma and misconceptions. Political ideologies and economic factors play a crucial role, particularly in the way people with dyslexia access diagnosis and services. For example, in Australia, the high cost of dyslexia diagnosis and treatment, along with limited government support, exacerbates social inequalities. Dyslexic individuals often face barriers to accessing essential resources, leading to long-term negative impacts on education, employment and quality of life.

Legal influences are also explored, particularly the role of the Disability Discrimination Act (DDA) and the Fair Work Act, in protecting individuals with dyslexia in the workplace. While there are legal protections in place, many workplaces still lack awareness of dyslexia, resulting in insufficient support and adjustments for employees. Raising awareness and promoting inclusive practices are seen as key to reducing workplace discrimination and improving job satisfaction and productivity for dyslexic individuals.

The section calls for greater societal awareness and support for people with dyslexia, particularly through legislation and workplace adjustments. The goal is to create a more inclusive environment where individuals with dyslexia can reach their full potential without facing systemic barriers.

KEY TAKE-HOME MESSAGES

Systemic Barriers: Dyslexia is often misunderstood and stigmatised at the societal level, creating barriers to support and inclusion. Political ideologies, cultural attitudes, and economic policies significantly influence how people with dyslexia are treated.

Late Diagnosis and Inequality of Access: Many individuals with dyslexia are not diagnosed until adulthood, leading to missed opportunities for early intervention. There are significant disparities in funding and access to services compared to other neurodevelopmental conditions like autism, contributing to social and economic inequities.

Financial Burden: The high cost of dyslexia assessments and interventions, coupled with limited government support, places a financial burden on individuals and families. This creates further challenges in accessing necessary resources for success in education and employment.

Impact on Quality of Life: Lack of early diagnosis and support can result in lasting consequences for educational attainment, employment prospects, mental health and overall quality of life for individuals with dyslexia.

Legal Protections: While laws such as the Disability Discrimination Act and Fair Work Act offer some protection, there is a lack of awareness and enforcement in workplaces, leading to ongoing challenges with discrimination and inadequate workplace adjustments.

Need for Greater Awareness: Societal and workplace awareness of dyslexia is essential for reducing stigma, improving support systems, and ensuring psychological safety for individuals with dyslexia, allowing them to perform at their best.

Equity vs. Equality: True equity requires providing resources and opportunities tailored to the unique needs of individuals with dyslexia, rather than offering the same support to everyone. Equity aims to level the playing field, ensuring individuals with dyslexia can reach their full potential.

Call for Action: The chapter urges for systemic changes in policy, funding, education, and workplace practices to ensure better support for individuals with dyslexia throughout their lives.

ANTI-DISCRIMINATION CASE STUDIES

Changes in job responsibilities, such as promotions, team dynamics involving new members joining or departing, and shifts in business strategy can pose challenges for all employees. However, these changes may be particularly difficult for individuals with dyslexia. It is important to clarify that we do not imply that employees with dyslexia should be excluded from promotion, on the contrary, they can thrive with appropriate workplace accommodations, training and coaching.

Nonetheless, when job roles evolve, previous strategies that were effective for them may not suffice in adapting to these transitions. For instance, a shift into a new position, the departure of a colleague who provided support with reading and writing tasks, the onboarding of a new team member who prefers written communication over verbal, or an organisational change that requires a faster work pace, can create stressful and vulnerable situations for individuals with dyslexia, when they are unable to disclose their dyslexia and access the workplace accommodations they need, as illustrated in the case study of Fatima..

Case study 1: Fatima - Food manufacturing manager.
Fatima, with a decade-long tenure in the manufacturing industry, holds a managerial position at a major food manufacturing company. Managing a team comprised mostly of women, she faces a challenge when a new male trainee, Philippe, joins her team. Six months into his tenure, Philippe lodges a formal complaint against Fatima, alleging that she deliberately withheld detailed instructions from him, requested in written format, implying discrimination based on his gender.

This discord escalates to a formal HR investigation, potentially jeopardising Fatima's job due to perceived bullying behaviour. In a pivotal moment, Fatima discloses her dyslexia; a condition she had never revealed before. Her training style, which had proven effective with previous team members, did not require extensive written documentation. The detailed instructions sought by Philippe were challenging for Fatima, due to her dyslexia, leading to a misunderstanding that culminated in his formal complaint.

Revealing her dyslexia to her employer, Fatima expresses shame and fear, explaining she had successfully managed her condition without issue, until now. She emphasises her reluctance to disclose her dyslexia earlier, driven by concerns about potential judgement and stigma. Fatima's emotional response underscores the personal toll of the situation, as she grapples with the fear of job loss and the embarrassment associated with the misunderstanding that led to accusations of sexism.

This case study illustrates the complexities that can arise during a change in job roles or changes in the workplace, where misunderstandings rooted in undisclosed conditions can lead to conflicts and formal investigations. It stresses the importance of open communication and understanding of diverse learning styles within a team, to prevent such issues from escalating to HR investigations.

Case study 2: Lucy – Bank clerk and the change of manager
Lucy, a bank clerk who openly shared her dyslexia with her initial team and manager, went beyond merely acknowledging her condition, she also provided insights into the specific challenges she faced, such as difficulties in spelling and pronunciation. Despite her candid disclosure, Lucy found herself working in an environment where she sensed that her team and manager lacked the necessary understanding, exhibiting limited tolerance for her dyslexia-related needs.

A significant shift occurred when Lucy was reassigned to a different area of the bank under a new supervisor. She disclosed her dyslexia to her new supervisor, and this time her supervisor, who was unfamiliar with dyslexia, took proactive steps. The supervisor undertook independent research to gain a better understanding of dyslexia and its implications. Following this, he engaged in a supportive dialogue with Lucy, expressing a commitment to collaborative problem-solving. He assured Lucy they would work together to develop strategies and implement adjustments that could support her in her role. Lucy felt empowered and truly understood.

Unfortunately, when this supportive supervisor left the following year, Lucy's positive experience took a downturn. As anxieties and concerns resurfaced, Lucy hesitated to disclose her dyslexia to her new supervisor. However, realising the importance of accessing the support she had previously received, Lucy eventually decided to share her condition. Regrettably, her new manager responded unsympathetically, stating, "This is a high-pressure industry. If you can't keep up, you should really think about another career." This dismissive attitude left Lucy feeling unsupported and undervalued, prompting her to contemplate the necessity of either moving to a different role within the bank or resigning. The positive feelings and sense of empowerment that had flourished under her previous supervisor quickly dissipated, in the face of this less understanding and unsupportive response.

This case study illustrates the complexities that can arise during a change in management and the lack of processes to support a staff member with a learning disability. It also demonstrates the negative impact on an employee when workplace adjustments are left to the manager's decision rather than it being a policy driven process applicable across an organisation.

3.2. THE EXOSYSTEM

Anything is possible when you have the right people there to support you.
Misty Copeland African American Ballet Dancer

The exosystem includes factors that have a direct impact on individuals' lives but are typically beyond their personal control (Bronfenbrenner, 2009; Hudson, 2014). This category encompasses traditional and social media, government agencies like the National Disability Insurance Agency, extended family, and the communities in which people reside. Often, these elements, whether intentionally or not, contribute to the creation of labels that define individuals within society through the development of administrative classification systems such as the label of dyslexia. In this section, we look at how dyslexia is diagnosed, who can diagnose dyslexia and the impact of this label, as well as the influence of social media, high profile celebrities and social entrepreneurs.

3.2.1. Communities

Under the exosystem is communities and the broader social and geographical environments where people live, which can influence social norms, resources and opportunities. Access to a diagnosis and early intervention greatly depends on what community you live in. You are more likely to access healthcare services living in a metro city compared to living regionally or remotely. However, there are still long wait times to access these services in metro areas. Wait times to access a dyslexia (learning disability) assessment vary across the country, from one month to six months in metro areas. For those looking for an autism or ADHD assessment in adulthood, the wait is even higher, being up to two years. All of this is distressing to hear when we know early intervention is key. For ADHD and autism, the assessments are not straight forward, needing allied health and medical professionals, while dyslexia assessment is conducted by allied health only. However, it's not as straight forward as you will see in this next section. So, let's look at what is involved in diagnosing dyslexia.

3.2.1.1. Diagnosing Dyslexia

The categorisation and application of diagnostic labels for neurodevelopmental conditions like dyslexia, ADHD, and autism has seen a markedly increased globally, particularly amongst adults [98, 167, 168]. Some would say that medicalised labelling has a greater overall impact on individuals than just to aid treatment of the specific condition affecting them. Work by Werkhoven et al (2022), identified four types of use for a diagnostic label, associated with neurodevelopmental conditions. These include science, therapy, administration and social contexts. In science, they provide medical labels of impairment, provide common language for health and research professions, and aid in data surveillance. Therapeutically, they guide interventions in therapeutic and pedagogical settings. Administratively, neurodevelopment conditions have a financial price tag attached to the label [168]. For example, in Australia, individuals with a diagnosis of autism are able to access funding under the National Disability Insurance Scheme (NDIS), and those individuals in the workplace with autism [80], ADHD and learning disabilities, aka dyslexia, can access a nominal fee annually for workplace accommodations, support and training [106, 169].

Often overlooked in discourse, is how these medical labels shape a person's self-identity, perceptions of others, and actions within the community [139, 170-172]. Nevertheless, diagnostic labels can offer some understanding and validation, that can provide insight into experiences and conditions, as can be seen among late-diagnosed autistic individuals and their families reported elsewhere [168, 173]. There are disadvantages to having a diagnostic label though, since it can also attain social bias.

As discussed, earlier dyslexia is recognised under the Diagnostic and Statistical Manual of Mental Disorders, Fifth Edition (DSM-5), which specifies that to diagnose a specific learning disorder, such as dyslexia, a clinical assessment is to be conducted to review an individual's developmental, medical, educational and family history. Test scores, teacher observations and responses to academic interventions are also considered. An individual must experience persistent difficulties in reading, writing, arithmetic or mathematical reasoning during their formal years of schooling [113]. To meet the criteria for diagnosis, the individual's current academic skills must fall well below the average range of culturally and linguistically appropriate testing of reading, writing or mathematics, and the individual must have received six months of evidence-based, high-quality instruction/intervention before a diagnosis can be made. Furthermore, the individual's difficulties cannot be better explained by developmental, neurological, sensory (vision or hearing) or motor disorders, and must significantly interfere with academic achievement, occupational performance, or activities of daily living [113]. The DSM-5 considers reading-underachievement, in relation to instructional opportunities, specifically through the response-to-intervention criterion. For individuals aged 17 and above, a history of documented learning difficulties can replace standardised assessment [113].

On the other hand, the International Classification of Disease (ICD-11) does not provide adult-specific criteria and determines underachievement based on cognitive ability [119]. Due to these differences, there are various ways of diagnosing dyslexia in adults. However, the DSM-5's response-to-intervention criterion may hinder diagnosis for individuals who have not had these opportunities, such as adults who are assessed later in life. As a result, concerns have arisen in the literature regarding the accuracy and consistency of dyslexia diagnoses in adults [174].

In countries like the UK, there are nationally recognised guidelines for identifying dyslexia in adulthood, within higher education environments [174]. These guidelines include a list of standardised assessments for cognitive achievement (such as the Wechsler Adult Intelligence Scale [175]), to ascertain discrepancies between high cognitive abilities and low literacy abilities (assessed by instruments such as the Wood-cock Reading Mastery Tests [176] [174]). The literature states that a major component of meeting the criteria for dyslexia is to score 1.5 standard deviations or more, below the mean on measures of reading and IQ/achievement tests in conjunction with the DSM-5 diagnostic criterion [43, 59, 174, 177].

However, in Australia there are no such guidelines to support clini-cians in assessing children, adolescents or adults [174, 178]. The DMS-5 diagnostic criteria are predominantly used to assess dyslexia, along with standardised assessments such as the Wechsler Adult Intelligence Scale and the Woodcock Reading Mastery Tests [178]. The lack of con-sistency and access to diagnosis, especially as an adult, can impede one's ability to access support and services within the workplace and beyond.

3.2.1.2. Who can diagnose us and how

Australian and international research has shown great variability in the age of diagnosis for individuals with dyslexia [15, 178-181]. This is at odds with other neurodevelopmental conditions, such as autism and ADHD, both typically identified in childhood, and often by an inter-disciplinary team [182, 183]. For some, if not most people with dys-lexia, this delay in diagnosis may result in the loss of critical early inter-ventions and support, including through the crucial years of schooling.

Sadly, Australia lags behind other developed countries regarding policies and practices for identification of dyslexia [184]. In the UK, qualified specialist teachers and educational/occupational psycholo-gists can diagnose dyslexia [185]. In Australia, educational psychol-ogists and/or neuropsychologists and speech pathologists are generally the professionals who assess for learning disabilities, such as dyslexia. Australian research undertaken by Sadusky et al. (2021) found that the way psychologists assess adults for dyslexia was not uniform with a variety of diagnostic standards used, and this is also generally compounded by a lack of national guidelines for operationally defining and diagnosing dyslexia within the adult population [178]. Access to these professionals can involve lengthy wait times and can also be financially prohibitive. As a result, many dyslexic people go undiagnosed or receive a late diagnosis. If diagnosis is delayed, the challenges that dyslexia creates in the school setting, can, and often does, continue into adulthood and the workplace.

International research shows great inconsistency in what constitutes dyslexia, how it is assessed, diagnosed and the age of diagnosis for individuals [15, 179-181, 186, 187]. Our research reflects and reinforces the current global ambiguity surrounding the definition of dyslexia, which may result in inconsistencies in dyslexia assessment and the risk of being diagnosed later in life. In Australia, as in many countries, age of diagnosis varies, and through my research, we are seeing a large proportion of the population getting assessed as adults. This is just too late! For many Australians, from the outset, the ability to access and gain a diagnosis of dyslexia and then follow up interventions, can be an ongoing challenge for children, young people and adults [123, 188]. In Australia, there is a lack of uniformity in the way individuals are assessed with a broad range of health professionals providing a dyslexia assessment. Other Australian research, such as Al-Yagon's work, also found variability by practitioners (e.g., psychologists, speech pathologists and general practitioners), and between Australian states and territories [123, 145]. Furthermore, there is no clear position across different disciplines about how dyslexia should be classified (e.g., learning difficulty, reading disorder, etc.) and little consistency in the application of diagnostic criteria found in the DSM-5. Additionally, while dyslexia is a complex bio-psychosocial condition, it is most often identified using psychometric assessments [123, 145, 178]. As such it has been found that some adults have been assessed for dyslexia using diagnostic tools designed for children. Further, several independent organisations and agencies in Australia also claim to provide dyslexia assessments, including pre-assessments and online self-diagnosis [189]. This lack of consistency in classification and identification can be costly, confusing and misleading, and makes access to an assessment even more difficult, highlighting fragmentation and gaps across the education and health sectors. Timely diagnosis and intervention are critical in enabling people with dyslexia to complete their education and to gain and retain employment [184].

3.2.1.3. Is a diagnosis important?

Getting a dyslexia diagnosis is important for several reasons. A formal diagnosis for some can be a revelation, as it can help with the ability to understand ourselves and validate why we have struggled and do things differently to others. It confirms that our difficulties with reading, writing and spelling are not due to laziness, lack of intelligence or a personal flaw, but rather a neurobiological difference.

It can enable us access to support, including interventions and accommodations. This is especially important for children in school. Schools can provide specialised instruction and accommodations tailored to their needs, such as extended time for exams, assistive technology, or access to a reading specialist. For adults, it means we can access workplace accommodations, such as assistive technology, more flexibility, such as working from home and other supports like one-to-one coaching. These accommodations can level the playing field and allow individuals with dyslexia to reach their full potential academically and in other areas of life. A diagnosis of dyslexia can foster self-awareness, helping individuals understand their strengths and weaknesses. It allows them to develop self-advocacy skills and communicate their needs effectively. By understanding their specific learning profile, individuals can explore different strategies and techniques that work best for them, increasing their confidence and independence.

Legal protections, as mentioned in earlier in Chapter 3, are so important. In Australia, dyslexia is covered under the Discrimination, Fair Work and Equal Opportunity Act [116, 120, 121] and a formal dyslexia diagnosis enables us to access certain legal protections and accommodations in educational and workplace settings. It can help ensure that individuals with dyslexia are not discriminated against and are provided with the necessary support and accommodations to succeed.

A diagnosis of dyslexia later in life, and missed opportunities for intervention, has the potential to impact a person's sense of self and leave them vulnerable to poor mental health and well-being over their life's trajectory [186].

As someone who was diagnosed at 27 years of age, and then had my first and hopefully only mental health break down, I can vouch for the problematic system we have and the implications for a late diagnosis. Yet, I was relatively young compared to the number of women I work with, who are being diagnosed in their late 30s, 40s and 50s. My own research has found 58% of diagnoses are in adulthood [98].

This means many children and young people are missing out on access to vital interventions that can support them as they transition into adulthood. If children and young people can't access services, we are setting them up to fail. Frankly, this is just not good enough. We don't want children growing into adults with literacy difficulties that could have been addressed in childhood. The long-term impact on mental health and well-being, and ability to participate fully in life, including education and then employment, should not be hampered because we can't get access to a diagnosis in childhood.

3.2.1.4. Access to mental health services

'...Psychologist response : So, her response to me telling her I was dyslexic and I do struggle with it, was she was literally like, 'I don't understand how you that would affect you and your mood. It shouldn't affect any-thing, and if it affects your work, then you should talk to them about it.' And I was like, 'Okay I'm not using this again.' It's not the first time I've had a counsellor or a psychologist say to me, 'Oh I don't understand why you have such a big issue with it,' or 'I don't understand why it affects you this way, it should just be something you can deal with...'
Research participant

As already mentioned, there is a lack of access to assessments to support the growing need of adults. Further, there is also a lack of access to the help they need. Adding to the frustration is the current lack of training for mental health practitioners (including psychologists and psychi-atrists) (MHP) on the dual diagnosis of dyslexia and mental health difficulties, and these are not neurodivergent affirming. When we talk about neurodivergent affirming, we are referring to an approach to understanding dyslexia, dysgraphia, dyscalculia, dyspraxia, autism, ADHD, Tourettes Syndrome, and other conditions that sit underneath this umbrella term. A neurodivergent affirming approach acknowledg-es that each neurotype comes with its own set of strengths, needs and challenges [190]. Instead of viewing these differences as conditions that need to be fixed or cured, this perspective emphasises acceptance, ac-commodation and support to help individuals thrive in a world that may not always be designed with their neurotype in mind.

Many dyslexics feel frustrated, let down and disappointed when they try and seek help for their mental health difficulties related to their dyslexia. Individuals with dyslexia in my research indicated that mental health practitioners frequently demonstrate a lack of understanding regarding dyslexia as a hidden disability, and its coexistence with mental health conditions. Many practitioners do not adopt a neuro-affirming approach in their practice, which limits their comprehension of the intersectionality and complexity of these individuals' challenges. These difficulties are often associated with past traumatic stress related to childhood, educational and workplace experiences. As well as potential co-occurring conditions such as ADHD and autism, alongside current issues related to anxiety, depression, and self-esteem. For many they may not even know they have a co-occuring neurodevelopmental condition as they have only had the opportunity to be assessed for dyslexia. For individuals with dyslexia, this knowledge gap can translate into inadequate support and a lack of tailored interventions to address both their learning disability and mental health concerns.

Presently, a critical issue is the absence of comprehensive training programs for mental health practitioners that focus on dyslexia as a disability and the enduring mental health difficulties that dyslexic individuals may encounter. There are a significant number of training programs now being developed for ADHD in adulthood, autism and neuro-affirming practices for these neurodivergent groups but nothing for those with dyslexia, which is why this book, research and the work we do at **re:think dyslexia** is so important. This is an urgent matter that needs to be addressed. Training needs to occur to address dual diagnoses of dyslexia and co-occurring mental health difficulties across different levels, including in universities and as professional development for psychologists and mental health professionals. This will ensure that future and current mental health professionals are equipped with the knowledge and skills to address the complex intersection nature of dyslexia and mental health. Ultimately, this proactive approach can lead to improved outcomes and a better quality of life for individuals navigating the challenges of dyslexia and its impact on their mental well-being.

3.2.2. Societal influences

The narrative of dyslexia in our community is significantly influenced by mass media, which also sits under the exosystem. The main two types of narrative identified through my work are ableist language and the use of labels. Labels are often perpetuated by social media, the media at large and those without lived experience. These narratives reflect and influence how communities think and understand dyslexia. A common belief is that dyslexia is about all the letters moving on the page, but you know this is not what it's about! So, what is *Ableism* and why am I talking about high profile celebrities? Well let's unpack this now.

3.2.2.1. Ableism and Labels

The language and the labels place upon us are examples of the societal context and how these can have a direct effect on us as individuals. Research demonstrates the inconsistency observed in the labels used to diagnose and characterise the challenges faced by those with dyslexia. Alongside the term 'dyslexia,' various descriptors such as 'neurodivergent,' 'disability,' 'learning difference,' 'learning preference,' 'learning disability' and 'learning difficulties' are being used to describe dyslexia [145]. Studies by Snowling (2020) and Wissell et al (2023) found that adults predominantly identified with and embraced the label 'dyslexia' more than any other term to explain their condition. The connection to the label of dyslexia remained strong during both their formative educational years and into adulthood.

Ableism is frequently referred to as a form of "social-level oppression" intricately linked with other systemic oppressions such as racism, sexism, classism, and heterosexism [191]. It intersects with the concept of intersectionality, acknowledging the multifaceted identities and experiences of individuals. Ableism is grounded in the idea that disability makes a person inferior, and that causes far too many to feel 'marginalised, discriminated against and ultimately devalued in this society' [192]. When we think of the different labels used to describe dyslexia, they are often imposed on us within the contexts of education, professional endeavours, and broader societal interactions, rather than being chosen by the individuals themselves. My research paper *"I hate calling it a disability": Exploring how labels impact adults with dyslexia through an intersectional lens. Under review:*, highlighted the presence of ableist language in workplace encounters, when colleagues who shared their dyslexia with colleagues and management, were met with comments such as *"you don't look dyslexic"*, *"what is it like to have an intellectual disability?"*, *"you can leave this meeting as you won't understand what we are talking about because you are dyslexic"*, *"you don't look dumb"*[145]. I had a manager once tell me she *needed a few drinks before reading my work,* and another tell me, *I knew something was wrong with you,* when I shared that I was dyslexic. Ableism can also be seen in the way people behave, such as speaking and talking really slowly, sending you lengthy emails or asking you to read lengthy documents, using all Capitals in text when you have said it is difficult to read, making statements like *I a must be dyslexic I can't spell* when you are not dyslexic and so on … you get the gist. I had a team member who would snigger when I asked how to spell a word.

Image 10. Charlotte

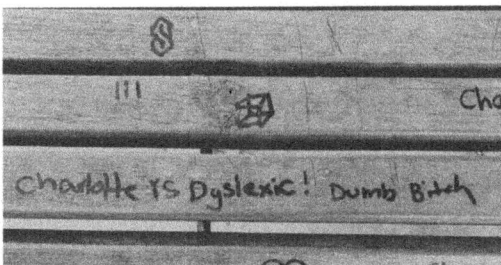

Take Charlotte as an example in Image 10. This was written on a park bench near my home. Charlotte could be your student, your employee, your child's friend. Do you think Charlotte is feeling very good about herself right now or into the future, or do you think Charlottee is going to go through life no matter how well she achieves with an underlying feeling of being dumb? I'll leave that for you to ponder. The concept often can be applied here, to identify acts of discrimination or prejudice evident, or perceived, towards the individual with dyslexia. These labels can adversely impact individuals' self-image, confidence and performance, perpetuating ableist assumptions and practices that build barriers and perpetuate inequalities for people with disabilities.

3.2.2.2. High profile dyslexics and the Dyslexia 'Superpower' Narrative

In the past decade, there has been a noticeable trend of celebrities openly endorsing dyslexia, which has served as a potent advertising and marketing strategy. Its primary aim has been to raise awareness about dyslexia and to highlight the numerous successful celebrities, entrepreneurs and scientists who also have dyslexia[145]. This has created a narrative within some parts of the dyslexic community, suggesting that some individuals with dyslexia hold remarkable abilities and talents. In my research, *"I hate calling it a disability," Explore how labels impact adults with dyslexia through an intersectional lens. Under review,* found that the concept of dyslexic superpowers resonated mostly with highly educated individuals who had reached the pinnacle of their careers [145]. It's worth noting that not everyone in the research attributed these superpowers directly to their dyslexia.

Conversely, most dyslexics did not identify with the notion of superpowers to describe their dyslexia. Instead, they viewed their experiences through the lens of a social model of disability, where environmental factors were seen as disabling elements, and their dyslexic difficulties made them feel disabled [145]. Interestingly, employers in my research recognised that when dyslexic employees had the appropriate workplace accommodations in place, dyslexia could be an asset in the workplace. Employers could identify specific strengths exhibited by dyslexic employees such as strong problem-solving skills, big-picture strategic thinking and seeing things differently than those who didn't have dyslexia [145, 193].

All dyslexics, regardless of their perspective on superpowers, identified the strengths and positive attributes they posed in and out of the workplace [145]. They felt that these strengths were often the result of developing strong compensatory strategies, such as problem-solving skills to get them out of having to disclose, perseverance in continuing to show up even when things were hard, self-awareness of their difficulties and their strengths and lateral thinking. Scholars like Goldberg et al. (2005), McNulty (2003), and Wissell et al. (2022b) have observed these qualities in existing research.

Yet the dyslexia 'superpower' narrative has become part of the cultural movement we are seeing globally, with the aim of emphasising strengths over deficits. Eide & Eide (2011), Beever's (2022) and *Dyslexic Thinking* (2024) are just some examples of this positive reframe. "*The Dyslexic Advantage: Unlocking the Hidden Potential of the Dyslexic Brain*" by Eide & Eide has leveraged this narrative travelling around the globe sharing their thoughts, whether rightly or wrongly. Eide proposes that around 20 per cent of individuals with dyslexia exhibit a distinctive learning difference that can be advantageous in various settings, [194]. They argue that dyslexic processing predisposes individuals to crucial mental functioning abilities, including three-dimensional spatial reasoning, mechanical aptitude, the capacity to recall significant personal experiences and the ability to comprehend abstract information through specific examples (Eide & Eide, 2011). The use of labels such as *superpower* can impact self-identity and societal attitudes. Acceptance of this label within the dyslexic community varies, highlighting the need for positive labels that reflect individual experiences without imposing limitations.

Made by Dyslexia, a UK-based charity, has launched global initiatives like "*The Value of Dyslexia: Dyslexic Capability and Organizations of the Future*," a report co-authored with Ernst & Young [195]. These efforts, along with their "*Dyslexic Thinking Campaign,*" aim to spotlight the unique strengths of dyslexic individuals, framing them as superpowers [145]. Recently, Dictionary.com recognised "*Dyslexic Thinking*" as a formal term, describing it as a problem-solving and learning approach characterised by pattern recognition, spatial reasoning, lateral thinking and strong interpersonal skills [196]. Additionally, the social networking platform LinkedIn has now included *Dyslexic Thinking* as a recognised workplace skill [145, 197]. Yet to date, we have not seen many professionals on LinkedIn, particularly in Australia, using the term *Dyslexic Thinking*. I feel there is still too much stigma attached to being dyslexic to showcase it on a professional site that may impact career opportunities. I have known some people who have added the *Dyslexic Thinking*, and then taken it off their profile because they have noticed less recruiters contacting them. Is this a coincidence? I'm not sure, but it may highlight the ongoing discrimination faced by those with dyslexia.

However, there are others who dispute the notion of dyslexia being a gift or superpower, as indicated in Lisa Moats' article dated April 26 2018, and there is a growing backlash from the dyslexic community. Contrary to the belief that dyslexia is inherently a gift, the current research suggests that problem-solving and creative abilities are not inherently more dominant in individuals with dyslexia [198]. Like all neurodevelopmental conditions, dyslexia is on a spectrum, and assuming an individual's dyslexia will automatically result in a set of gifts can be misleading, considering the lifelong challenges that many dyslexics face.

Viewing dyslexia through the intersectional framework, we can start to see how power, privilege and oppression can play in how individuals and society perceive dyslexia. This perspective, however, has the potential to exacerbate social inequalities and give rise to subsequent social issues [199]. The characterisation of dyslexia as a superpower can be seen as a privilege, a descriptor employed by those with influence and financial means to articulate their dyslexic abilities or disabilities. However, those individuals who don't see their dyslexia as a superpower but more of a disability or a hindrance may start to feel isolated, marginalised and disempowered, potentially leading them to avoid seeking help [145]. We are starting to see some backlash on social media platforms now. These types of ability labels may cause dyslexics to feel higher levels of anxiety and stress, leaving them to feel inadequate or left searching for a fictitious superpower. My latest research emphasises the significant variance in perspectives between dyslexic individuals, employers, experts and the media, which warrants further research. If employers recognise dyslexic individuals and their strengths as valuable assets to the organisation, with skills increasingly relevant in today's evolving work environment, rather than concentrating solely on their challenges, it will create a more inclusive working environment where everyone thrives. Emphasising a strength-based approach and labels resonates with dyslexics, rather than using the labels of superpowers, which may mitigate the risk of further marginalisation and fragmentation within this population.

I personally do not see my dyslexia as a superpower, nor do many other adults I interviewed through my research. At best, I see it as a hindrance to my day-to-day quality of life; at its worst, it can be a crippling disability that leaves me embarrassed, frustrated and in a state of flux. I can't see in 3D, I'm terrible at art and I don't resonate with any of the other 'so-called' gifts and/or superpowers that we are supposed to have. However, I have learnt to live with my difficulties, and it has not limited me in any way, shape or form in achieving what I have wanted to achieve, because I have had the right support. Of course, not everyone has the opportunities I have had. If anything, my dyslexia has pushed me harder, it has given me more focus and a drive to constantly do better and to accomplish more. Is that a superpower? We will talk more about resilience and perseverance in later chapters.

CONCLUSION

In summary, the chapter highlights some of the systemic barriers at the exosystem level that significantly influence those who are outside the dyslexic control. These elements include the way the medical model diagnoses and classifies dyslexia and who can diagnose it. This chapter also discussed why it is so important to be able to access a diagnosis. It helps people gain a better understanding of themselves, and it protects them under different laws and legislation. Finally, it also highlights the lack of neurodivergent-affirming services and trained mental health practitioners who understand and can provide appropriate interventions for a dual diagnosis of dyslexia and mental health conditions, which is often overlayed with the complexity of co-occurring difficulties. Whether the individual is aware of them or not.

Another area under the exosystem was the role of societal influences, including the use of labels, both positive and negative labels, placed on those with dyslexia. Additionally, this chapter showcased the role of mass media, high profile celebrities and business owners are playing on the perception of dyslexia within society. The prevalence of ableist

language and the "superpower" narrative, reflect a shift from the deficit model we have seen and know to a more positive way of framing
dyslexia. While some view dyslexia as a unique advantage, others see
it as a source of significant personal and professional challenges. This
discrepancy highlights the need for further research into the way dyslexia is seen, understood and represented across society and, more importantly, the lived experience of dyslexics included in these narratives.

KEY TAKE HOME MESSAGES

Exosystem Influence: The exosystem includes external factors like media, government agencies and community resources that significantly
impact individuals' lives, particularly through administrative classification systems and diagnostic labels.

Diagnostic Criteria Variation: Diagnosing dyslexia involves diverse criteria, with the DSM-5 emphasising clinical assessments, academic underachievement, and a response-to-intervention criterion.
Discrepancies between DSM-5 and ICD-11, especially in adult diagnosis, raise concerns about accuracy and consistency.

Global Disparities: Worldwide, there is great variability in dyslexia diagnosis, notably in the age of diagnosis and the professionals
involved. While the UK has national guidelines for adult diagnosis,
Australia lacks uniformity, leading to delayed or missed diagnoses and
continued challenges into adulthood.

Impact of Late Diagnosis: Delayed dyslexia diagnoses, often occurring in adulthood, hinders access to crucial interventions. This delay, coupled with the lack of consistent assessment standards, contributes to ongoing struggles in education and employment, impacting
mental health and overall well-being.

Importance of Diagnosis: A dyslexia diagnosis is crucial for
self-understanding, dispelling misconceptions and acknowledging

neurobiological differences. It enables access to tailored support, accommodations in education and the workplace, fostering self-awareness, self-advocacy and legal protections.

Lack of Neurodivergent-Affirming Practices: Mental health practitioners often lack training in dual diagnoses of dyslexia and mental health issues, leading to inadequate support. A neurodiversity-affirming approach, recognising diverse neurotypes, is essential for fostering understanding and providing effective care.

Societal Influences and Ableism: Media portrayal and societal attitudes, including ableist language and stereotypes, affect how dyslexia is perceived and experienced. High-profile endorsements of dyslexia as a "superpower" can both raise awareness and perpetuate unrealistic expectations.

Complex Intersectionality: Dyslexics face challenges in mental health services due to practitioners' insufficient understanding of dyslexia's complexity, intersectionality and links to past traumatic experiences. This knowledge gap results in a lack of tailored interventions to address both learning disabilities and mental health concerns.

Need for Comprehensive Training: There is a pressing need for comprehensive training programs for mental health practitioners to address dyslexia as a disability and its enduring impact on mental health. Integrating such training into professional education can ensure empathetic care, improved outcomes and a better quality of life for individuals with dual diagnoses.

Need for Support and Accommodation: Access to appropriate support and accommodations is essential for individuals with dyslexia to thrive academically and professionally. Legal protections and tailored interventions can play a crucial role in leveling the playing field.

Call for Action: Addressing the gaps in diagnosis, support, and understanding of dyslexia requires a concerted effort from healthcare providers, educators, policymakers and society to ensure that individuals with dyslexia receive the recognition and support they need.

3.3. THE MESOSYSTEM

The mesosystem encompasses those elements of society that have a more immediate relationship to the individual. For example, a person's family, school, workplace, friends, peers and regular health professionals are all part of the mesosystem [9, 94, 153]. These is a lot to cover in the mesosystem, my head is spinning, so I have broken it down into smaller chapters for you to make it easier to digest.

3.3.1. Negative childhood experiences

There is strong evidence linking negative early life experiences to poor mental health and well-being [200-202]. Although research has been conducted to investigate the co-occurring difficulties of mental health and autism [203], limited Australian research has been conducted into the links between negative childhood experiences within the education system for people with dyslexia and the impact of these on psychosocial well-being in later adult years. We hear a lot from the autistic community about the trauma caused by the medical model including misdiagnosis, mistreatment and over/wrong medication, all which have had a lasting negative impact on their community [204]. Although dyslexia sits under the medical model for diagnosis, we don't seem to link the medical model to traumatic experiences. However, we do see links between trauma and the education sector. Many with dyslexia have faced educational trauma in their formative years, with this trauma being carried into adulthood as post-traumatic stress syndrome, which aligns my research with international findings, if somewhat small [205]. I think this not only needs to be acknowledged and addressed but also investigated and evaluated. This is not about blame. I believe when

I was at school, teachers did the best they could with the tools and skills they had. But in 2024, we know better, and things must change because we are still seeing young people traumatised by the education system. Despite perceived positive educational outcomes in Australia, my research found, for some students, traumatic experiences relating to their dyslexia did occur during their formative educational years into secondary school education. This led to elevated levels of emotional distress, and stress occurred due to bullying from peers and teachers, including name calling such as *dumb, stupid, lazy* and *idiot*, being asked to read and spell words aloud in front of the class, as well as having to write on the blackboard/whiteboard in front of peers, and being publicly humiliated and singled out for spelling and maths mistakes in front of the class, having to attend special education classes with children who had intellectual disabilities, high needs autism and behavioural issues. My research also highlighted dyslexic students having to work twice as hard than their non-dyslexic classmates to learn the same concepts, causing significant mental fatigue trying to keep up with peers, work tasks, studying for tests, completing assignments and homework activities all contributing to the traumatic experience some endured at school. These experiences can even cause dyslexics to engage in internalising behaviours for both girls and boys to *like* feeling stupid, dumb, inadequate, anxious, angry and frustrated as children and young people, consequently having a profound impact on their self-esteem and self-worth [206]. Some young people, in particular boys, tend to turn to externalising behaviours by bullying others, getting into fights, disengaging from school and getting into trouble. Whereas externalised behaviours for girls, could appear as becoming perfectionists, people-pleasing and always wanting to do the right thing, making it hard to pick up their underlying difficulties [206]. In other instances, some children and young people may turn to things they are good at and can focus on, like sport and the arts. Regardless, many individuals with dyslexia experience traumatic events in childhood that leave an imprint on their soul as they progress into adulthood. The ongoing lack of understanding and awareness of dyslexia, especially in secondary school, is a major concern. There has been a significant focus and funding on other neurodevelopment conditions, and again, now in 2024, we are still seeing dyslexic children left behind and traumatised, leading to disengagement in education; we can't learn if we are scared, anxious and stressed. And this has a flow-on effect into adulthood. There is one thing you must remember, when it comes to dyslexics, we never forget; we never forget how we were treated in school, it is scorched into our brains forever! These imprints can play out in different ways as we will discuss now and in the section on *social and emotional well-being* where ongoing stress can lead to post-traumatic stress syndrome.

3.3.2. Education and qualifications

To date, there is only a handful of local research [31, 207-209] that examines how dyslexia impacts educational attainment across vocational training and higher education. The only Australian study we could identify was from the Australian Temperament Project; a life-course longitudinal study of psychosocial development [31]. This study investigated early adulthood education and employment outcomes related to reading difficulties and behavioural problems in childhood, although not specifically or solely relating to people with dyslexia. The rest [207-209] focused on the experiences of adults with dyslexia within vocational training and higher education settings, rather than educational attainment outcomes.

Reading difficulties have been found to be a unique risk factor for poorer educational outcomes, with co-occurring problems highlighted in Chapter 2 (such as ADHD, dyscalculia and dysgraphia), significantly increasing this risk [31]. It is therefore anticipated that participants in this research would have lower than average educational attainment compared to the general population. Contrary to this assumption, the participants across my research were highly educated, more so than the national population average. Most participants (79.74%) had attained an education level of Year 12 and above, compared to only 68% of the general population (Australian Bureau of Statistics, 2019). One explanation for this difference in results could be that educational opportunities have increased across the education and higher education sectors over the past two decades, as a better understanding of dyslexia as a disability has emerged [107, 207, 210, 211] [212]. Access to reasonable adjustments for people with disability in the education and higher education sectors, including those with dyslexia, are now mandated globally through laws and legislations [116, 157, 213] . However this is fraught with difficulties due to funding and diagnositc requirments for TAFE and Universities, as well as the absence of standardisation..

People with dyslexia in education and higher education, can now access assistive technology, have additional time to complete assignments and sit exams, and use other adaptations, like audiobooks and speech to text, and text to speech software [212, 214, 215]. These adjustments may explain why many of the cohort in my research had completed secondary school and gone on to undertake vocational training and higher education. However, this does not explain how a considerable number of participants in my research, who were diagnosed with dyslexia as adults, were still able to gain vocational training and post-graduate qualifications. Without a diagnosis of dyslexia in their formative years, these participants would not have had access to early interventions and/or reasonable adjustments to support their learning disability. So what enabled them to be so successful? We will find out in the coming chapters!

3.3.3. Relationships and social connections

As young people move into the developmental stage of adulthood and begin to interact more directly within the mesosystem, they begin to face a different set of experiences, challenges and complex demands. Regardless of a diagnosis of dyslexia, adulthood presents several new and varied experiences and adjustments for all individuals. For many adults with dyslexia, there may be additional challenges based on their childhood and adolescent experiences that can further complicate navigating these demands. These challenges include vocational training, higher education, managing at work, socialising and building relationships, late diagnosis and interconnection with other neurodivergences [73, 216-218]. As we know, these challenges can lead to elevated levels of psychological distress and be associated with lower income, lower educational attainment, and unemployment [31].

Building relationships and social skills is complicated for everyone; there are times when all of us think we could have done better, said something differently, been more kind or considerate. However, for those with dyslexia, building and maintaining relationships can be hard at times. Why you might be wondering? We don't usually associate relationship challenges with dyslexia. However, building social competence requires skills in being able to initiate and maintain social relationships, encompassing cooperation, trust and good communication [219]. It's the communication aspects where we can be let down and we accidently let others down as well. Let's look at some of the areas that those with dyslexia, including myself, may struggle with verbal and written communication, building friendships, the impact of trauma to understanding jokes, puns, sarcasm and more!

Several international scholars, as far back as 1995, have explored the social interactions of adults with learning disabilities/difficulties [57, 220, 221]. These studies have identified a subgroup of dyslexic individuals who demonstrate successful social interactions, whereas others encounter challenges in developing and maintaining relationships. Despite some successful social interactions among certain dyslexic adults, others may experience social and emotional difficulties throughout their lives due to the impact of dyslexia on their communication skills, self-esteem and overall psychological well-being [220-223]. My research noted that the trauma of past humiliations, feelings of social embarrassment and isolation, and the fear of making mistakes, re-emerged for dyslexic adults in social settings later in life. Those with dyslexia can struggle to manage and follow conversations and understand jokes, leading to feelings of being socially awkward. For me, I would just follow the social cues and laugh when everyone else does, but my husband knows me too well, and will turn around and say, *"you don't get it do you,"* and I say *"no,"* so then he tries to explain. Often, I am left feeling dumb and insecure about myself because I don't get these social cues, and this can chip away and erode confidence over time.

Research now strongly supports the notion that friendships and positive relationships are protective factors in reducing the risk of poor mental health and well-being - for all people. However, several studies have highlighted that those with dyslexia can have difficulties developing friendships, collegial and intimate relationships [139, 224-226]. To my knowledge, there is no research looking into the technology tools that we use to communicate with, and one that could be causing lots of issues, is the online dating arena. My research revealed that individuals utilising online dating platforms expressed concerns regarding the potential for online shame stemming from their spelling errors. The challenges of navigating the dating process in an environment that necessitated written communication caused distress and apprehension.

The impact of dyslexia on intimate relationships is an area that requires further exploration. Alexander-Passe, found in his research, that individuals with dyslexia often conceal their difficulties, only revealing their challenges when compelled to do so – a decision influenced by the potential risk of jeopardising a successful relationship. Dyslexics may encounter specific communication difficulties in their relationships, ranging from struggles in reading social cues and pronouncing lengthy words to introducing unconventional elements into conversations. The disruption of routines can lead to panic, and tasks may be performed in the wrong sequence, causing the dyslexic partner to be perceived as socially inept [227]. I know my mum would get so frustrated when my dad would randomly change the topic part way through a conversation. She always thought he was just being rude, until we read Alexander- Passe's work!

Kjersten (2017) observed that some dyslexics tend to gravitate towards partners that are high-functioning individuals and who can complete tasks that dyslexics may struggle to undertake. Non-dyslexic partners express surprise at the extent to which their dyslexic partner relied on them to complete day-to-day activities [57]. Adding to Kjesten's work, Alexander- Passe also found the non-dyslexic partners can get frustrated by their dyslexic partner's perceived inability to perform simple day-to-day tasks, such as crafting a shopping list, taking phone messages, managing finances, or forgetting where they have left items like car keys, prompting many non-dyslexic partners to assume responsibility for day-to-day activities within the home [227]. My work also found, that as those with dyslexia transitioned into adulthood, their reliance on family was reduced as they became more dependent on intimate partners and peers to support day-to-day activities and to manage in the workplace.

Kjersten's (2017) study also found that when a dyslexic's partner encounters difficulties in their relationship, it can trigger heightened emotions, which may also relate to past traumatic experiences from childhood, particularly in relation to negative school experiences, such as shaming and bullying, and challenges with developing peer relationships [228-230]. This emotional response often leads to feelings of shame and can hinder their ability to regulate emotions effectively, as processing feelings can be particularly challenging for some dyslexics [57]. Consequently, they may resort to various coping strategies. Difficulties in emotional expression, typically arise from feeling overwhelmed, leading to responses such as withdrawal or emotional outbursts. It is important to recognise that both reactions can occur, rather than just one or the other causing a communication breakdown within relationships [57]. If a non-dyslexic partner becomes critical of a partner with dyslexia, this can lead to self-criticism, anxiety and depression, leading to poor overall mental health and well-being [57]. Without a comprehensive understanding of their partner's neurodiversity, it is easy for them to misinterpret certain behaviours, such as withdrawal or frustration. Such misunderstandings, can exacerbate existing emotional pain and feelings of inadequacy that dyslexic individuals may already experience due to past challenges with failure and shame.

Effective communication is a critical area where dyslexic individuals may struggle, impacting their ability to form and maintain both casual and intimate relationships. Misunderstandings, difficulties in reading social cues and challenges in written communication, such as those encountered in online dating, can lead to feelings of inadequacy and social isolation. It is important to note, that for some dyslexics, achieving and sustaining these relationships often requires significant effort and understanding from both partners. Additional co-occurring conditions such as autism and ADHD can add further complexities to relationships. The emotional toll of these ongoing struggles can contribute to higher levels of psychological distress leading to poor mental health. Therefore, it is crucial for society to foster greater awareness and understanding of the broad ways dyslexia can affect individuals and relationships. This is particularly important for mental health practitioners and relationship counsellors to understand, when working with dyslexic individuals and couples.

Through my podcasts and Facebook Lives, I have interviewed a number of experts, couples and individuals who all spoke openly about the challenges of developing and maintaining friendships and intimate relationships. Coupled with this (pardon the pun!) is my research which also highlights the challenges we face. But why might this be? Well I could give you plenty of personal anecdotes about the ups and downs I have had with my siblings and partners along the way, and my now husband. It's not just our writing that is at times impaired, but it can be our mouths as well! Work weighted by Alexander-Passe and Kjersten highlights how dyslexics can get words mixed up when we get stressed or anxious; our brains may stop working as we try to process what is being said and then decide how to respond. There are a number of different things that can be going on in our brains! Many of us can, and do, have successful relationships, all relationships are hard, but it doesn't mean dyslexics can't enjoy and have fulfilling intimate relationships!

3.3.4. Family support and other relationships

'...My parents were terrific, in that they didn't set expectations about what I would do or be interested in. Whatever I wanted to do, I never felt it was a 'bad' thing to do, as they were always encouraging me. That led to a sense of validation in my choices. I might have struggled with other people judging my academic capability, but my parents never focussed on that. It was a huge positive...'

SHAE WISSEL

Research participant

Parental relationships play a role in protective factors that support dyslexic children as they grow and learn. Parenting is hard work whether your child is dyslexic and/or has other neurodivergences, or they are not. It places pressure on our relationships, finances and our ability to work at a level we are used to. It also squeezes our time ... what time? And if we are neurodivergent then it can add an additional layer of complexity, as we navigate a world that demands we be more organised, meet health appointments, learn how to navigate the horrendous online system of Centrelink and MyGov ... and all these things we need to manage, while making sure we meet the needs of our families. It's exhausting enough - without being neurodivergent. As a mum with a toddler, I have never felt as tired as I do now. As mentioned earlier, as our children grow up, the chances of them having dyslexia is high, and there is not a lot of research or evidence-based information to help us navigate as a dyslexic/neurodivergent parent.

When a child is diagnosed with a disability such as autism, hearing impairment and intellectual disabilities, some parents often experience grief, related to the loss of hopes and expectations [231, 232]. Along with grief are feelings of social isolation, guilt, anger and fear of the future - for themselves and their child [233, 234]. For some, there will be guilt that their genetics have been passed on to their child ... and then what if they face all the struggles you did? So much to unpack!

If you already know you are dyslexic, then you probably already have many great strategies that support you, and you know where to get the help you need. I know if my daughter is dyslexic, then I know where to go and what we will need to do. But not all parents have knowledge of what services are available and this can hamper their ability to receive the right help. Knowledge is important and can play a crucial role in helping parents and children, when moving in the right direction to obtaining their child's diagnosis [235]. Insufficient knowledge about dyslexia can hinder parents' ability to come to terms with the diagnosis and support their child effectively. As parents seek to educate themselves about dyslexia, they can transform their initial negative perspectives into a more positive outlook [235]. Understanding dyslexia can be achieved through various resources, including school support, local support groups, through health professionals and peak organisations **such re:think dyslexia**, the British Dyslexia Association, Auspeld or Learning Difficulties Australia, just to name a few. Supportive family dynamics are essential, as they can empower children with dyslexia to complete their education and pursue higher learning opportunities [95, 236]. Positive paternal involvement is particularly beneficial in assisting children in understanding their diagnosis. Research indicates, that adults with dyslexia who reported having supportive parents, experienced higher self-esteem compared to those without familial support [229]. Parents who actively educate themselves can also foster positive educational experiences and teach their children essential skills, such as self-advocacy, from an early age.

The literature suggests that the presence of family support (or lack thereof) can be a protective influence in self-esteem, can help adults cope with emotional difficulties and can reduce the negative experiences associated with dyslexia [229, 236]. Familial support, including those of siblings, can also be very helpful. But research on sibling support for people with dyslexia is limited and I could only find a handful of research papers [237, 238]. It is important to understand the impact of sibling relationships on self-esteem can be both positive and/or negative for a dyslexic person. This has been illustrated through the large body of research that has been conducted on autism and or ADHD, [239-242]. You could assume there are positive correlations between this research and the experiences within the dyslexic community. If only we had more research!

'...It affects my parenting. One of the things I've really struggled with is teaching my kids how to read. When I had to start teaching them phonetics and how to break down a word and chunking - I can't do that. And being a single parent as well, that's absolutely impacted their reading ability. My anxiety over them being able to cope at school [has] impacted them...'

Research particpant

But what about the dyslexic parents? What can be done for them? What can be done for parents like me??

Some of the challenges for parents with dyslexia were highlighted in Alexander-Passe's work and through my research. Alexander-Passe (2015) found that some parenting styles of dyslexics indicate a deep-seated aversion to matters related to school, particularly interactions with teachers, reflecting their own negative experiences. My research also found the impact of dyslexia on parenting, including challenges communicating through technology, such as texting, feelings of inadequacy when they couldn't read to their children or help them with their homework, and how they perceived the impact of their own anxieties about their dyslexia and educational trauma. This all impacted on their children's academic success. Further research needs to be undertaken in this area and the impact of late diagnosis of parents on the family, trying to learn about yourself, your struggles and strengths, while supporting your own dyslexic, neurodivergent child, is a lot, and you shouldn't have to do it all on your own.

As previously mentioned, the financial cost of assessment and early intervention can be a significant barrier for many families. Supporting a child with dyslexia requires ongoing literacy support, including regular sessions with a speech pathologist and tutoring, from a young age through the transition into secondary school. Dyslexia is a lifelong difficulty with costly interventions attached, demanding considerable time and energy from parents to navigate and advocate for their child's needs. Seeking external help for students outside of school, creates additional financial burden for parents. If improved training of teachers was prioritised for assisting students with learning difficulties, this might negate the need for parents to get help elsewhere. Teacher training can get lost in the myriad demands of teaching requirements. The complex challenges for teachers and schools needs to be addressed, so that dyslexic children do not fall through the cracks.

Consequently, parents and families bear the burden of covering the financial costs of support and advocating for their children. This situation leads to many children falling through the gaps, not due to their parents' efforts, but because of societal barriers that hinder success. To address this issue, we must create more equitable solutions for those with dyslexia and their families. The added complexities of managing dyslexia can strain family relationships and compromise mental health and well-being. If one parent is dyslexic the added pressure of trying to support their dyslexic child is huge. We are asking too much of parents and families, and it is clear that systemic changes are necessary to provide better support for families dealing with dyslexia.

Now if you have heard my podcasts or heard me speak, you will know what an important role my mum, sister, aunty and other family members, friends and my husband have all played in supporting me and enabling me to be where I am today. I miss my mum so much every day, and the unconditional love and support she provided me. My mum would proofread all my assignments at school and university, and when I was in the workforce, she would read emails, reports and other materials I needed proofread. And I'm not alone! Through my research I found similar stories to mine. Many children and adults with dyslexia relied heavily on their parents, particular their mums, who played a major role in facilitating their educational progression, by helping them complete academic tasks, advocating for their needs, and seeking alternative support when they felt the school system was not meeting this.

3.3.5. The pros and cons of technology when communicating

There is no research I could find outside of my work, that discusses the difficulties of communicating in adulthood, using technology. Recent advances in technology have created complications - for some of us. Now don't get me wrong, I love ChatGPT and couldn't survive without Google maps, Siri and, of course, Grammarly, but when trying to communicate with friends, family and work colleagues using different types of written tools, such as social media, online dating forums, emailing, messaging apps and text messaging, things can get tricky. My work found, for the better or worse, that all these advances require and make public our written communication skills. Many people have been trolled online and ridiculed because of their spelling and grammar mistakes on social media, making it a source of embarrassment and exclusion from participating in what, are now, socially acceptable ways of communicating and interacting with others. It can be a source of stress, hampering relationships, both personal and work-related.

Communicating through text messages between family and friends can leave some of us feeling vulnerable and worried about being misinterpreted or misconstrued. We now have the research to back it up. I know from personal experience, and have been told my text messages and emails are harsh, direct and to the point, without any niceties or what I would call *fluff*. This has always been a point of contention for some of my friends and my siblings! At times it has caused major arguments, and it has always frustrated me, because to me, clearly there is still such a lack of understanding and awareness at the mesosystem between friends, families, and the broader community, about how we dyslexics communicate. I feel there is no leeway for this disability. It is such a point of frustration for those who are not dyslexic, but would we get frustrated if someone was partially deaf and they couldn't follow the conversation? No, we would be considerate and adjust the way we speak or the environment to ensure they could hear. But I feel for many dyslexics, this isn't happening as we are left feeling disheartened and, at times sad, that the people who are supposed to love and care for us the most are the ones who get the most frustrated. Okay rant over, I love you siblings!

When we consider all of the above – limited and inconsistent recognition of support for dyslexia as a disability; changing definitions of disability; inconsistent policies and practices for the identification of dyslexia; lack of awareness of dyslexia and its impact in educational institutions and in the workplace; and, the difficulties that can arise within relationships when one partner has dyslexia – we can see how some or all of these factors may influence how people with dyslexia see themselves as individuals.

3.4. CONCLUSION

This chapter highlights the major lack of research that has been undertaken until now looking at the impact of negative early life experiences that are carried through into adulthood. The work demonstrates the strong link between negative early life experiences and poor mental health and well-being, which is particularly concerning for those with dyslexia, who often endure emotional distress, bullying and a lack of understanding within educational settings. Despite those with dyslexia achieving significantly high educational outcomes, with many completing undergraduate degrees in Australia, many faced educational trauma that affected their social and emotional well-being well into adulthood.

The financial burden associated with assessments and early interventions, further complicates the situation for families and adults. Supporting a child with dyslexia demands ongoing literacy support and substantial parental advocacy, often without adequate assistance from educational institutions and the government. This imbalance highlights a societal barrier that needs to be addressed, to prevent children from falling through the gaps.

Family support plays a pivotal role in the lives of dyslexics. Parents, particularly mums of dyslexics, played a significant role in ensuring their children succeed. Yet the emotional and financial toll is significant on families, and more resources, research and support systems are needed to help these families and children thrive. By addressing the educational, social and emotional challenges faced by dyslexics, we can work towards creating a more inclusive and supportive society. The next chapters will delve deeper into the specific ways in which individuals with dyslexia navigate their mental health and well-being through the microsystem lens.

KEY TAKE-HOME MESSAGES:

Impact of Negative Early Life Experiences: Negative early life experiences, particularly within the education system, significantly affect the mental health and well-being of individuals with dyslexia. Bullying, emotional distress and lack of understanding can leave lasting trauma.

Financial Barriers: The cost of assessments and early interventions poses a substantial barrier for many families. Ongoing literacy support and parental advocacy are crucial but can be financially and emotionally draining.

Systemic Educational Challenges: Many schools and secondary education institutions are inadequately trained to support dyslexic students. This lack of support often forces parents to bear the full burden of advocacy and financial costs.

Higher Education Achievements: Despite these challenges, many individuals with dyslexia achieve higher education levels, possibly due to increased awareness, reasonable adjustments, and supportive technologies. However, systemic support needs improvement.

Social and Relationship Struggles: Dyslexia impacts social interactions and relationships. Negative school experiences and communication difficulties can lead to social isolation and strained relationships. Support and understanding are essential for improving social well-being.

Crucial Role of Family Support: Family support, particularly from parents, plays a vital role in the success and well-being of individuals with dyslexia. Dyslexic parents face unique challenges in supporting their children, highlighting the need for more resources and support systems.

Need for Systemic Change: There is a clear need for comprehensive and systemic support for individuals with dyslexia and their families. Addressing educational, social, and emotional challenges is crucial for creating a more inclusive and supportive society.

Future Directions: Further research and advocacy are necessary to understand and address the complexities faced by individuals with dyslexia. This includes exploring educational and vocational achievements, relationships, and the critical role of family support in greater depth.

3.5. THE MICROSYSTEM

The Bronfenbrenner theory put forward that the microsystem represents the most immediate and smallest environment in which children reside. This applies to adults as well. Consequently, the microsystem encompasses the surroundings of one's home, workplace, peer group and community. Interactions taking place within the microsystem typically involve personal connections with family members, classmates, teachers and caregivers. The way these groups or individuals engage with children plays a crucial role in shaping their development. When interactions and relationships are characterised by nurture and support, it is more likely that a conducive developmental environment is created. Bronfenbrenner suggested that many of these interactions are reciprocal in nature; the way children respond to individuals within their microsystem will also influence how these individuals reciprocate their treatment of the children [146, 153].

Ok, we just looked at some of the protective factors and risk factors from childhood through to adulthood that can impact someone who has dyslexia. It's been a long tough read and/or listen so far and I hope you can hang in there to finish off one of the most important parts of the book; our social and emotional well-being. This last section draws on the microsystem and summarises how all these different interconnected intersections of our lives have a role in how we develop as children into adults. These interconnections also impact on our mental health both positively and negatively. The associated difficulties of having dyslexia and other neurodivergences impact on mental health in several ways, across employment, socio-economic status, physical well-being, social and community connections, and psychological and emotional well-being. Not everyone who has dyslexia has problems in all these areas, nor are they experienced all at once. If you are dyslexic, you probably already know which area, or areas, are the ones you need some support in.

There has also been an increase in the number of psychological disorders stemming from the workplace, including depression, post-traumatic stress disorder and anxiety. Psychological disorders may occur due to mental and emotional fatigue, bullying or harassment, trauma and excessive or prolonged work pressures. In Australia, there is a void in the literature concerning the link between negative childhood experiences within the education system that have a flow-on effect into adulthood. However, the research is clear that early life experiences can considerably influence people's health and well-being, education, employment, interpersonal relationships and community and economic engagement [243]. Stressful events at any point in the life course may have important consequences for psychosocial and physical functioning in later life [244]. The experience of dyslexia, whether diagnosed or not, will have a considerable impact on an individual's sense of self-worth, and on their values and belief-systems throughout adulthood [245, 246].

3.5.1. Trauma and Post Traumatic Stress Syndrome Disorder

For now, what seems to be missing from previous literature in Australia, is that there appears to be a significant amount of chronic stress and mental fatigue experienced by people with dyslexia, that develops in childhood and may be over and above that experienced by the average person. Although stress is a normal human reaction affecting all people, my work found that, from an early age, many people with dyslexia appear to be in a continuous state of stress. This aligns with other neurodivergent conditions, such as autism, where from a young age, neurodivergent children are under substantial amount of stress compared to their peers, leading to mental health difficulties in adulthood [247]. Chronic stress has been known to negatively alter the brain's development, especially when we are children and particularly in relation to motivation, memory, thinking, reasoning and emotional regulation

[248]. Stress responses can elicit different emotions and behaviours and could contribute to the 'fight, flight or freeze' behaviours described by some participants in my research (e.g., school truancy and anger).

Those who are exposed to chronic stress and traumatic experiences are at risk of post-traumatic stress disorder (PTSD). International research highlights the link between other neurodivergent conditions, such as autism, with PTSD [247, 249] and suggests over 80% of individuals with PTSD suffer from at least one additional disorder [250]. Work by Haruvi-Lamdan et al (2018) found a strong intersection between PTSD and Autism, the occurrence of traumatic stress among individuals with autism and the perspectives on traumatic events, particularly within the social context [249]. There is minimal exploration of dyslexia and trauma. Alexander-Passe's study (2015) demonstrates that people with dyslexia may feel: *"the sudden exclusion from their peer group; intense anger from a teacher or parent; physical bullying at school; the realisation that something unrecognisable is wrong (maybe realising that they are not normal or do not learn normally), being called stupid, lazy etc."* [205].

Although my research did not directly investigate the link between childhood trauma and PTSD, it was evident that some individuals appeared to experience PTSD related to their childhood experiences, which caused significant challenges in adulthood. These challenges included diagnosed anxiety and depression disorders, some of which were being treated with medication, as well as substance misuse. In relationship and workplace settings, individuals with dyslexia could appear oversensitive, overreactive and highly emotional when faced with difficult situations or feedback, both positive and critical. They also faced difficulties forming relationships, ongoing health problems, challenges in the workplace and managing day-to-day activities. This research strongly supports local and international findings that children, adolescents and adults with dyslexia and other co-occurring difficulties, face considerable mental health issues originating in childhood that can lead to PTSD in adulthood.

3.5.2. Self-concept

If you think about the child who doesn't get access to an assessment or early intervention in primary school, how do you think their sense of self develops overtime, if they are continuously made to feel different from their peers and others around them, and/or if they are bullied, discriminated against and made to feel less than others? You could see they could start to develop a negative sense of self from a young age that follows them through into adulthood. Imagine how the person feels by the time they get into adulthood. Do you think they are living their best lives? Are they like Charlotte, who we discussed earlier, that has felt dumb and stupid all her life?

As we transition from being a child to an adult, the development of our self-concept evolves. How we see ourselves and the world in which we live, is influenced by our childhood experiences and the environment we grow up in [251]. For people with dyslexia, the struggle to attain functional literacy skills can lead to the development of low self-esteem and low self-confidence [97]. A study by Palombo (2001) found that people with learning disabilities may develop negative self-narratives (stories one tells themselves), to make sense of their emotional and personal experiences. Those who feel they are not good enough or that they are a failure, may have difficulties accepting their disability/difficulties and the functional struggles they will have throughout their life [252].

Understanding how negative childhood experiences affect psychosocial well-being in adulthood, is pivotal to the way we support children, young people and adults. When an individual with dyslexia is faced with ongoing negative experiences, these appear to reinforce feelings of stress, shame, frustration and embarrassment and create an internal paradigm of negative self-beliefs, inadequacy, anxiety and fear associated with their dyslexia. This can lead dyslexics to be at risk of developing a negative self-concept through their early childhood experiences and is linked to educational trauma, adverse relationships with peers and a lack of support within the family unit. The literature highlights that internalising negative feelings can affect one's self-esteem [206, 253, 254]. When children are labelled, and those labels are associated with negative connotations, this can result in low self-esteem. Low self-esteem has been associated with feelings of inadequacy and frustration [172]. Researchers have found that negative childhood experiences, such as adverse comments from teachers, can have a devasting impact on the way students perceive themselves and their academic self-concept. These negative impacts on self-esteem can be carried into middle age as those with dyslexia continue to compare themselves with other adults even when, as adults, they are successful [97, 114, 245]. Education trauma mentioned earlier can also be carried through to adulthood, leading to many hiding their dyslexia and leaving them feeling little self-worth. This underscores the importance of providing adequate support and understanding to children with learning difficulties to foster positive self-esteem and overall well-being.

3.5.3. Mental health and well-being

We have already touched on social and emotional well-being earlier and now we will look at the mental health conditions that dyslexics can develop when unsupported. Research by Brunelle found that 56% of dyslexic adolescent students were found to have anxiety and depression, compared to their non-dyslexic peers. When they looked at socioeconomically vulnerable students, they found that 74% scored higher on anxiety and depression measures than their non-dyslexic peers [101]. If we look through an intersectional lens, we can see the role socioeconomic status plays as a protective factor or risk factor for dyslexic individuals and the impact it can have on mental health and well-being.

Anxiety is a common mental health condition that can be intertwined with dyslexia. Dyslexic individuals may experience anxiety related to their difficulties with reading and writing. For example, the fear of being called upon to read aloud in the classroom or in the workplace, or the anxiety surrounding writing, can all be sources of significant stress. This anxiety can manifest as performance anxiety, social anxiety or even generalised anxiety disorder, affecting both their academic and social lives. The constant worry about making mistakes or not meeting expectations can be emotionally taxing, adding to cognitive fatigue and mental overload.

Depression can also be a consequence of dyslexia-related struggles. The persistent challenges and frustrations associated with dyslexia can lead to feelings of hopelessness and sadness over time. Individuals with dyslexia may feel overwhelmed by their difficulties and isolated from their peers, which can contribute to the development of depressive symptoms [102]. The sense of not fitting in or not being able to achieve their potential in the workplace, and life in general, can weigh heavily on the mental health of those with dyslexia, potentially leading to clinical depression.

My research used the Warwick-Edinburgh Mental Well-being Scales (WEMWBS), a standardised tool we used to look at the overall well-being of adults with dyslexia in Australia. It was not surprising to know, that in our sample, mental health and well-being was significantly compromised [98] compared to the general population in Australia and internationally [4, 255]. Specifically, those with dyslexia reported lower self-confidence, poorer self-esteem, and more mental fatigue [98]. As discussed earlier, negative self-perceptions can have a lasting impact on mental well-being, potentially contributing to the development of mental health issues. Low self-esteem and a lack of confidence can be significant barriers to achieving personal and academic goals, further exacerbating feelings of frustration and helplessness.

These scores of the WEMWBS are supported by the results from my other research studies looking at the workplace [155, 256], where dyslexics reported feeling mentally exhausted, unsafe to disclose their disability (due to potential discrimination), socially isolated and unable to be their true authentic self in the workplace. Considering the internalising and externalising factors, it may be inferred that these factors are instrumental in comprehending why individuals with dyslexia, despite having achieved a high level academically and being employed, are still experiencing notably lower levels of mental health and well-being, as well as lower overall life satisfaction ratings compared to the general population.

While dyslexia itself is not a mental health disorder, it is a risk factor for lower levels of mental health and well-being. Poor self-concept, low self-esteem, anxiety and depression are some of the mental health challenges that can emerge because of the challenges and frustrations associated with dyslexia. Recognising these potential intersections is essential for providing appropriate support and intervention to individuals with dyslexia to help them manage their emotional well-being and succeed in various aspects of their lives. Further research is needed to unpack which of these factors, if any, play a greater role than others and the role of specific types of interventions and support that may help to buffer these stressors.

3.5.4. Conclusion

In examining the protective factors and risk factors associated with dyslexia from childhood to adulthood, it becomes evident that dyslexia can significantly influence various facets of mental health and well-being. Dyslexia's impact extends across career well-being, financial stability, physical health, social connections and emotional well-being, with individuals facing challenges in diverse areas.

Research consistently highlights that individuals with dyslexia experience lower overall well-being, heightened mental fatigue, and are more susceptible to anxiety and depression, with a disturbingly elevated risk of suicide attempts. Anxiety and depression are identified as common mental health challenges intertwined with dyslexia, manifesting as performance anxiety, social anxiety and generalised anxiety disorder. The persistent challenges associated with dyslexia can contribute to feelings of hopelessness and isolation, potentially leading to clinical depression. The overall mental health and well-being of adults with dyslexia in Australia, as measured by the Warwick-Edinburgh Mental Well-being Scales (WEMWBS), indicates significant compromise compared to the general population.

Exploring the potential intersection of dyslexia and Post-Traumatic Stress Disorder (PTSD) underscores the role of chronic stress in altering brain development. While dyslexia's link to PTSD is less explored than other neurodivergent conditions, research indicates a significant association. The potential impact of childhood trauma on adults with dyslexia is highlighted, showcasing challenges such as anxiety, depression, substance misuse, emotional sensitivity and difficulties in various life domains.

Bronfenbrenner's microsystem theory emphasises the importance of immediate environments, including home, workplace, peer groups, and community, in shaping individuals' self-concept. For individuals with dyslexia, negative childhood experiences can lead to the development of a negative self-concept, perpetuated by feelings of stress, shame, and inadequacy, impacting self-esteem even into adulthood. Workplace-related psychological disorders, overrepresentation in the criminal justice system and the scarcity of literature addressing negative childhood experiences in the education system, further compound the challenges faced by those with dyslexia.

While dyslexia itself is not classified as a mental health condition, the challenges and frustrations associated with it can significantly impact individuals' mental well-being. Recognising the intersections of poor self-concept, low self-esteem, anxiety, depression and socioeconomic vulnerabilities, are crucial for providing tailored support and interventions. There is a need for further research to explore the effectiveness of specific interventions in buffering stressors and enhancing emotional well-being. Understanding these complex dynamics is essential for fostering a supportive environment that enables individuals with dyslexia to thrive in various aspects of their lives.

KEY TAKE-HOME MESSAGES

Diverse Impacts Across Life Domains: Dyslexia has multifaceted effects on mental health, influencing career well-being, financial stability, physical health, social connections and emotional well-being. Recognising these diverse impacts is essential for providing holistic support.

Elevated Mental Health Risks: Individuals with dyslexia face heightened mental health risks, including lower overall well-being, increased mental fatigue and a doubled likelihood of experiencing anxiety and depression. Disturbingly, the risk of suicide attempts is 46% higher in individuals with dyslexia compared to the general population.

Workplace Challenges: Dyslexic individuals are susceptible to psychological conditions in the workplace, contributing to depression, post-traumatic stress disorder and anxiety emphasising the need for tailored support.

Childhood Trauma's Long-lasting Impact: Negative childhood experiences related to dyslexia can have enduring effects on individuals' mental health, contributing to conditions like anxiety, depression, substance misuse and emotional sensitivity in adulthood. Addressing childhood trauma is crucial for comprehensive support.

Self-concept Development: Dyslexia significantly influences the development of self-concept, with negative childhood experiences leading to stress, shame, and inadequacy. Understanding the impact on self-esteem is vital for interventions that promote positive self-narratives and self-worth.

Anxiety and Depression as Common Challenges: Dyslexia is associated with anxiety and depression, stemming from challenges with reading, writing and the fear of social and academic expectations. Identifying and addressing these challenges is crucial for promoting mental well-being.

Measurement of Mental Health: Standardised assessments, such as the Warwick-Edinburgh Mental Well-being Scales (WEMWBS), reveal compromised mental health and well-being among adults with dyslexia in Australia. Tailored interventions and support are essential to address lower self-confidence and higher mental fatigue.

Supportive Environment and Interventions: Recognising the complex dynamics of dyslexia's impact on mental health is crucial for fostering a supportive environment. Further research is needed to explore the effectiveness of interventions in buffering stressors and enhancing emotional well-being.

Holistic Understanding for Holistic Support: To provide effective support to individuals with dyslexia, it is imperative to adopt a holistic understanding that considers the interconnectedness of various life domains and addresses mental health challenges comprehensively.

RESOURCES

There are a huge number of resources you can find so we are listing just a few to help you on your journey of discovery and understanding. You can find more information at re:think dyslexia.com.au. If you found any of this content distressing, please seek support:

- Lifeline on 13 11 14
- BeyondBlue counsellor on 1300 22 4636
- NEAP Neurodivergent Employment Assistance Program on 1800 13 6327

Organisations supporting neurodivergent adults:

- re:think dyslexia
- ADHD Australia
- Neurodiversity Hub
- Untapped Holding

Books, podcasts and support

- Work by Neil Alexander-Passe
- Invisible Disabilities, Visible Success (Dio Press)
- The Successful Dyslexic-Identify the keys to unlock your potential (Sense Publishers)
- Dyslexia and Mental health
- Dyslexia and Depression: The Hidden Sorrow: An Investigation of

DYSLEXIA

Cause and Effect (Psychiatry-theory, Applications and Treatments)

Work by Jane Kjersten

- Dyslexia and intimate relationships: Disconnection, disunion or a call to embrace difference?
- Understanding and working with dyslexia in individual and couple therapy Implications for counsellors and psychotherapists
- **Dear Dyslexic Podcast** on your favoured podcast platform and subscribe, rate, and review.

Relevant Dear Dyslexic podcast episodes:

- Episode 68: From Classroom to Career: How Dyslexics Pass, Mask, Cope and Succeed with Dr Neil Alexander Passe.
- Episode 66: The Business Case for Inclusion: Dr. Jamica Nadina Love on Cultural Add.
- Episode 65: The Impact of Late Dyslexia Diagnosis: A Conversation about art, resilience and self-discovery with Kim Percy.
- Episode 52: Dyslexia and Workplace Law with Barrister Ben Fogarty.
- Episode 47: with Pennie Aston CEO of GroOops and dyslexia and counselling
- Episode 44: with Jane Kjersten on dyslexia and relationship
- Episode 38 Intimate relationships with Jane Kjersten

Counselling Support
- Jane Kjersten

- GROOopS in the U.K.
- Dr Malvika Behal

Peer support
- Dear Dyslexic closed Adult Facebook group
- Dear Dyslexic PhD and dyslexic researcher

Part Two
THE JOURNEY INTO THE WORKPLACE: A DYSLEXIC PERSPECTIVE

The right of persons with disabilities to work on an equal basis with others; this includes the right to the opportunity to gain a living by work freely chosen or accepted in a labour market and work environment that is open, inclusive and accessible to persons with disabilities.
Convention on the Rights of Persons with Disabilities

Are you still with me? As you can see, the journey into adulthood is tough for many dyslexics. It's a rocky, and at times, unforgiving road. It leaves us with layers of armour to protect us from a world that doesn't understand us, at times doesn't help us, and can make us feel undervalued and unappreciated.

I feel exhausted, sad, disappointed and yet, filled with hope, because I know change is coming, and although the journey into adulthood is hard for everyone, you can now see the layers of complexity faced by dyslexics. And so much more can be done now, and into the future, to mitigate and reduce these difficulties.

That's where the hope comes in. Unfortunately, it's at the end of this book but that's not the end of the journey! After reading this, for many of you, the journey will just be beginning; from self-discovery to awareness to normalising what is happening to us and around us. Now the next section of the book is hard to read as well and there may be tears, sprinkled, hopefully, with some humour, but at the end the gold threads that keep the hope burning will shine though ... yay!

So, get your favourite beverage of choice; possibly a coffee, tea or gin. I would suggest some good brie cheese, make yourself a little antipasto platter, get comfy and settle in. If you are dyslexic and neuro-divergent, hopefully these chapters add to your toolbox for managing life, in and out of the workplace. If you are an employer, manager, leader, in HR or anyone else. get curious and get ready to learn about how you can support young people and adults in the workplace to thrive.

Andiamo (Let's go)

Chapter 4

DYSLEXIC EMPLOYEE PROFILE

4.1. DYSLEXIA DIFFICULTIES

There is a lot to get through in the next section, and I hope you are ready to reflect, learn and implement, so you can build and retain a strong workforce. In the resource section, you will find a neurodivergent workplace audit that can help you to review your workplace strengths and areas that can be improved. But first let's look at the general difficulties someone with dyslexia might have in the workplace, from when they enter the labour market through to late career. We will be learning more about the difficulties across the employment life cycle in the upcoming sections based on what my research found, but for now, let's look at the general workplace challenges a dyslexic may have. And remember dyslexia is on a spectrum and can affect people differently; not everyone will have all these difficulties listed below.

4.1.1 Dyslexia and the spike profile

Graph .1. Dyslexia and the spike profile

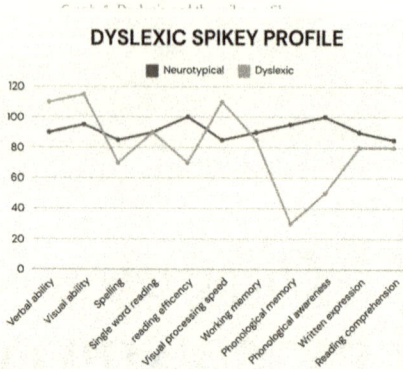

DYSLEXIC SPIKEY PROFILE

■ Neurotypical ■ Dyslexic

(Graph showing values: 120, 100, 80, 60, 40, 20, 0 on y-axis; x-axis labels: Verbal ability, Visual ability, Spelling, Single word reading, reading efficency, Visual processing speed, Working memory, Phonological memory, Phonological awareness, Written expression, Reading comprehension)

If you can remember, early on we talked about the areas of strength and difficulties that might present for a dyslexic. This can be presented visually through a spikey profile, as seen in Graph 1. You have may have heard this term used for other neurodivergent conditions.

So, over the coming chapters remember that those with dyslexia will have areas of difficulties, but also areas of strength, that you as a manager, leader and employer can harness in your workplace!

Workplace Difficulties

As we learned earlier, dyslexia affects the mechanisms involved with reading, which has a flow-on effect to writing and maths. But how does this present in the workplace? As a dyslexic, manager, leader, employer what might you be noticing? Let's take a deep dive now into how dyslexia can present in the workplace.

4.1.1. Literacy skills

4.1.1.1. Reading

'…I miss keywords a lot of the time; I'll miss all sorts of written information that sits on a page. I do a lot of detailed reading, and if I miss it, it can often have consequences, or it means I've got to be slower…'
Research participant

Individuals with dyslexia face significant challenges in reading and writing, which are often crucial in various workplaces. Dyslexics have difficulties with reading comprehension, fluency and speed, which slows everything down, such as reading and comprehending reports, case notes, medical reports, building and floor plans, policies and procedures, job manuals and emails. The list is endless, but the point to remember, is that reading will take extra time compared to their colleagues [256, 257]. Extensive reading requirements can lead to feelings of cognitive overload and mental fatigue. You may notice some dyslexics are strong in the morning and by afternoon slow right down, as they become more and more fatigued, especially if they don't have the right workplace accommodations.

For some people, reading might look like the letters are moving on the page. A common misconception is that this happens for everyone, and it DOES NOT. For me, the letters *b* and *d* appear to flip on the page when I read a sentence, especially when I am tired. This means when I get to the end of a sentence, it doesn't make sense, so I go back and re-read it, and that slows me down, but I still comprehend the information; it just takes me longer. If there are numbers in a sentence, as in research papers, my reading slows down even more. At university, I would read a few pages of a journal article and fall asleep! But don't worry; there are plenty of tools to support reading in the workplace, and it can be as simple as using Microsoft Immersive Reader or Speechify.

4.1.1.2. Writing Skills

'... We do have a lot of written work, which, again, I sort of use the same words all the time, so it makes it easier, but it's frustrating that I can't express what I want to say. I think you also sometimes seem a bit less intelligent because you use basic words. I want to use the big words in my head, but I can't put that because I don't know how to spell it...'
Research participant

When reading skills are impacted, this can lead to difficulties with learning how to spell, with a flow-on effect with grammatical structuring of sentences, leading to poor sentence structure. Sentences may be missing small connecting words like *to, on, in,* morphemes including suffixes, such as *es, ed, er* and *ing* and past, present and future tense confusion. [8, 14, 112]. This means sentence structure becomes confusing. Although we might be able to verbally articulate what we are trying to say, putting it on paper can be completely different. This can also impact vocabulary, as we struggle to spell the words we would like to use and then must simplify our writing to a level that doesn't fully demonstrate our skills and capabilities. For example, if someone struggles to spell *excellent,* they might simplify the word with one that is easier to spell, such as *great.* When I couldn't spell a word, people would suggest I look it up in the dictionary. For those young people who don't know, a dictionary was a large book that had all the different words and how to spell them. But if you don't know the beginning of the word, such as, 'Does *three* starts with *th* or *f*?' then it's hard to look it up in the dictionary. Despite the employee's meticulous efforts in editing and reviewing, errors will persist due to difficulties in proofreading. Dyslexics struggle to identify mistakes, and just like suggesting they use a dictionary, asking them to read their work aloud is also not a helpful solution.

At least now, AI tools are here and can significantly improve how we read and write. When I used to work in an office, I would ask my team member (I would get laughed at) how to spell a word, and during COVID, I would ask my husband. Now, I ask Siri, and Siri knows how to spell everything for me, including Italian words. Now, I am more independent and autonomous with my writing, something that would never have happened even five years ago. Thanks to Steve Jobs (he was dyslexic!) Tools like text-to-speech, Grammarly or the Hemingway App can be valuable aids in proofreading and editing for all dyslexic employees, but also those where English is their second language, those who might not have finished school and/or if writing isn't their strength. These are universal tools that can help everyone. Further details on these tools will be discussed in later chapters.

4.1.1.3. Numerous Skills

As we discussed earlier, there is a link between dyslexia and numerous skills, and for some individuals, their maths can be impacted, although they don't have dyscalculia. This is because they may have difficulty reading and comprehending math instructions, retaining numbers in their short-term memory and/or getting numbers mixed up and confused. For example, I struggle to see multiple zeros in a spreadsheet or document and get my thousands, millions and billions confused. I had a manager once correct my report because I had one billion dollars when it should have been one million! For me, it is like reading a foreign language. Although I love a good spreadsheet sometimes, I find it difficult to read and comprehend when there are lots of big numbers. However, there are lots of people I know who are dyslexic and work in finance, and they have no issues with numbers or spreadsheets.

4.2. EXECUTIVE FUNCTIONING DIFFICULTIES FOR DYSLEXICS

Workplaces commonly demand efficiencies in areas that dyslexics will struggle with outside of reading and writing. Executive functioning refers to a set of cognitive processes that include working memory, flexible thinking and self-control. These skills are crucial for managing tasks, organising information, and regulating behaviour. Barlett and Mood (2010) identified three areas that sit under executive functioning that might not appear obvious to a manager:

Working memory is needed in tasks such as remembering more instructions, numbers and sequences, taking minutes/note taking, following a discussion. Dyslexics have difficulty holding and manipulating information in their mind, which can affect their ability to hold and retain information.

Example: Notetaking, following multi-step instructions given verbally and keeping track of deadlines. Please don't make dyslexics be the note takers! This is not our skill set and it is exceptionally hard for us to do, especially if we are self-conscious about our handwriting and spelling. Again, everyone is different, I actually have good working memory for some tasks but not for others.

Organisation skills: Managing time, organising tasks, prioritising responsibilities, and meeting deadlines require effective planning and organisation skills. However, individuals with dyslexia might struggle with these aspects due to difficulties in processing information quickly. This can result in frustration, missed deadlines and a sense of being overwhelmed by tasks leading to a sense of mental exhausting and cognitive overload [257, 258].

Example: Finding it challenging to create a coherent schedule or to-do list and sticking to it.

Working to speed with accuracy: A dyslexic employee may have to choose between working quickly and knowing that there will be a lot of errors, versus working meticulously and carefully but missing set deadlines [257].

Example: Working speed is reduced when reading and/or writing an email.

Task Initiation and Completion: Difficulty with starting reading and/or written tasks which in turn, often leads to procrastination. This can also affect the ability to see tasks through to completion.

Example: Delaying the start of a report because of the uncertainty on how to start writing it … so we stare at the blank page for ages.

4.3. VERBAL COMMUNICATION

A major difficulty that can present itself in the workplace is the ability to process verbal information especially if it is in rapid succession, with multiple steps. Individuals with dyslexia might require additional time to process and internalise information. When they do not have enough time to process the information, it can lead to misunderstanding, which can lead to mistakes being made, affecting the individual and the team [259, 260]. In one-on-one interactions and group settings, verbal communication can be difficult if someone feels unprepared and/or 'put on the spot.' This may lead to some dyslexics having trouble rapidly recalling words, figures or information. It may also take them longer to process and respond to verbally to a verbal question or instructions. This can lead to a breakdown in communication where the dyslexic may hesitate or use word substitutions. They may struggle to articulate their ideas, leading to misunderstandings and inefficiencies. It is a bit like when we are pressured when communicating in relationships, as we discussed earlier. They may become flustered and stressed. From a manager or colleague's perspective, this may look like the dyslexic employee is incapable of understanding the work or cannot think independently. However, they need more time to process and articulate the information. When they don't have the time, expressing thoughts coherently and confidently can become a source of anxiety, potentially hindering effective workplace communication and collaboration [110, 257].

4.4. COGNITIVE OVERLOAD EQUALS MENTAL FATIGUE

'...I realised for the first time – I was struggling quite a lot, and it was affecting me quite severely. It meant I wasn't able to make my normal KPIs, as everyone else was; I was taking a slower time. I realised I was getting quite sensory overloaded as well, which was something new to me; I can't actually recall having that issue before. And I was just struggling in general, it was making me feel quite unhappy, uneasy, making me fear going to work and also made me quite question my own career path as well...'
Research participant

What is cognitive overload? "Cognitive load theory, also known as working memory load, refers to the amount of working memory resources an individual uses when engaged in a cognitive task" [261]. Cognitive overload is a state of mental exhaustion due to the limited capacity of working memory, which can affect performance due to increased demands placed on working memory which can lead to feeling of stress [262, 263]. Cognitive overload can affect anyone, but it seems to be a common phenomenon within the dyslexic and other neurodivergent communities when engaging in mentally demanding tasks that relate to their condition. There is not a lot of research on the impact of cognitive overload at work across neurodivergences. Yet, in my research, many participants talked about ongoing feelings of cognitive overload, leading to a sense of overwhelm and mental fatigue during their school years and in and out of the workplace. As discussed earlier, those with dyslexia can have trouble with working memory, so it's easy to see how they might become overloaded more quickly. When I explained to one of my mentors that I was feeling completely overwhelmed, she said *you are feeling discombobulated*, and she was right! I just couldn't get my "shit" together. As soon as she said that I felt a weight lift off my shoulders! For those with dyslexia, cognitive overload can feel like intense mental effort, and that leads to stress by continuously engaging in tasks that require significant cognitive resources such as reading, writing tasks and staying organised. At times, while writing this book, I felt significant cognitive overload and mental fatigue because I have a writing disability as well as a reading disability! It's not an excellent combination for an author, but I do it because the joy outweighs the overload most days!

What might cognitive overload look like for someone?

- **Difficulty Concentrating:** Trouble focusing on tasks or maintaining attention.
- **Mental Sluggishness:** Slower thought processes and difficulty processing information in particular relating to reading and writing tasks.
- **Memory Issues:** Forgetfulness or difficulty recalling information
- **Reduced Problem-Solving Ability:** Challenges in making decisions or solving problems effectively.
- **Increased Irritability:** Heightened emotional responses or frustra-

tion.
- **Feeling of sensory overload** – unable to cope with the sounds, lights or environment around them
- **Physical Symptoms:** Headaches, muscle tension or general feelings of tiredness.

When the brain is overwhelmed, it becomes exhausted, resulting in mental fatigue. Mental fatigue can lead to job burnout and significant mental health problems, which we will discuss in Chapter 7. Managing cognitive overload and mental fatigue involves taking breaks, chunking larger and or harder tasks into smaller tasks, and understanding how you work best so you can tackle complex tasks first or start small and build up. Everyone is different but looking at ways to reduce cognitive overload and mental fatigue is really important, and it starts with acknowledging that you may need support with some tasks, so you don't feel discombobulated! Build in enough rest, I love a good afternoon nap, maintaining a healthy lifestyle, and, in some cases, seeking professional help may be needed. We will discuss this further in Chapter 8: Workplace Accommodations that can help reduce cognitive overload and Chapter 9: Looking After Yourself as a Dyslexic Adult.

4.5. COPING STRATEGIES: SOME CALL MASKING, SOME CALL PASSING

'...I always went to the job early to set up myself and everything. It takes me more effort than most people to do things. I would come in early, stay late, skip lunch, etc. That seemed to annoy a lot of people. I don't understand why, but it did. I remember one time I was counting for myself. I would count through ways to make sure it was accurate. I had to work extra hard. Then they look at you and say, "Well, if you can achieve that,

then there's no problem with you. You don't have a disability. Or you don't
have learning disabilities." And that's the balance. I do. I work really
hard. And it's made me into a perfectionist person...'
Research participant

Within the neurodiversity community, the concept of *masking* is frequently discussed, as well as the negative impacts this can have on mental health. Masking is a term initially used in the autistic community
and refers to coping strategies that they use to hide or downplay their
autistic traits to conform to societal norms, such as mirroring facial ex-
pressions that wouldn't come naturally to them and forcing themselves
to make eye contact [264]. In the context of dyslexia, you might hear
us use the terms 'masking', 'passing', 'coping strategies' or 'workarounds.'
In his work, Neil Alexander-Passe talks about dyslexic passing rather
than masking. People with dyslexia often find themselves continuously
navigating decisions about when, where, why, and how to disclose their
dyslexia or whether to pass as neurotypical, presenting an appearance
of being *able-bodied* [138]. Passing refers to the act of hiding a particular aspect of one's identity - such as a disability, race, gender identity, or
sexual orientation - to appear as part of a more socially accepted group
[265]. In the context of dyslexia, passing involves concealing or moder-
ating the difficulties associated with dyslexia to present as neurotypical
or as someone who does not have a learning disability. This can be
done to avoid stigma, discrimination or misunderstanding. However,
passing, like masking, can lead to emotional stress. Although it makes
us good at problem-solving so people can't discover we are dyslexic, it
requires constant effort and energy to hide our true, authentic selves.
The decision to conceal or reveal our dyslexia can shape how we view
ourselves and how we are perceived by others, impacting our confidence and sense of belonging in various environments and affecting

self-esteem, confidence and social relationships [138]. It also means we are expending significant energy to appear neurotypical and cover up difficulties, often leading to feelings of cognitive overload, mental exhaustion, and fatigue and can lead to job burnout [138]. Examples of passing and coping strategies that dyslexics might use include sending work in and out of their workplace to have it proofread and checked, (yes that was me with my mum) emailing information to their phone to use AI tools that are blocked on their work computer and then emailing the information back once they have fixed it, or 'listening' to it, coming in to work early, working through lunch or working back late to keep up with their workload, not volunteering to do certain activities, such as reading aloud, writing on a whiteboard or taking notes in meetings, a reliance on colleagues to do tasks or to fix things they have difficulty with. You can see how this could lead to cognitive overload and mental fatigue.

Recognising and understanding the signs of passing or using coping strategies is essential for creating environments where not just neurodivergent employees but all employees can bring their whole selves to work without the need to conceal or adapt. We will discuss this in further detail in the chapter 5: Disclosure. By alleviating the pressure to mask and pass we can create inclusive environments where everyone feels valued for their unique strengths and perspectives.

When the work environment changes

A change at work is often difficult for everyone, but for dyslexics, there is an added layer of complexity. For dyslexics, there are three changes in the workplace that can be most difficult, including a change of environment, change of job role and change of manager. A dyslexic employee may be working exceptionally well within their current coping strategies and do not feel there is a need to disclose or share their dyslexia because the strategies they have in place are working well and they are performing well. When one of the three changes occur, their current strategies may no longer work or meet the changes that have occurred. Examples of change could be when a new manager comes in and introduces new systems and processes that requires the dyslexic employee to have a high level of reading and writing comprehension, change in job role that requires more reading, writing and organisation skills or the environment changes where you go from working at home efficiently, to an open planned office there it's hard to concentrate. This can result in their dyslexic difficulties becoming more pronounced as they may feel exposed and vulnerable [193, 256, 257].

4.6. LACK OF AWARENESS AND UNDERSTANDING.

Through my research and work, the largest obstacle that dyslexics had to face and overcome was the significant lack of awareness and understanding within organisations from colleagues, management, leadership and executives. At an organisational level, there was a disconnect between different departments' understanding of dyslexia and how to support dyslexic employees across HR and or People and Culture, DEI teams, Work Health and Safety and then the line manager. This issue stems from dyslexia not being understood as a disability and the different ways that it could affect individuals including misconceptions about it not being a disability, that dyslexia only affected reading skills, managers thinking because they knew someone who was autistic, or they were neurodivergent children, they understood what it was like for a dyslexic adult. This lack of awareness can be observed throughout the employment life cycle, as we will explore in the following chapters. Consequently, this leads many dyslexics to conceal or pass their dyslexic difficulties, prohibiting them from accessing the required workplace accommodations and then being able to work to their strengths. Let us now look at what these strengths are and how you could leverage them to create high-performing teams that feel psychologically safe and can achieve their optimal performance.

4.7. DYSLEXIA STRENGTHS: PERSONAL RESOURCES

We have just looked at all the different barriers that can impact someone with dyslexia in the workplace when they are not supported. When they are supported, their whole world is transformed, and they can bring their best, true, authentic selves to their workplace … yay!

As we touched on earlier, there is some controversy surrounding dyslexia and its strengths when labelled as a superpower. Everyone has strengths whether you have dyslexia or not. As we see the rapid advancements in technology around the world, some of the strengths identified by dyslexics could become more and more in demand [266]. A strength-based approach supports personal and organisational development that focuses on identifying and developing an individual's strengths, rather than their difficulties. This approach recognises that everyone has unique strengths and abilities which can be harnessed to achieve their goals and improve their performance. This approach is based on the belief that people are more motivated and engaged when they are doing what they are naturally good at, and when they feel valued and appreciated for their contributions. Focusing on strengths can help individuals develop a positive self-image, build confidence and improve their overall well-being. Additionally, it can enhance teamwork and collaboration by leveraging the strengths of each team member and creating a supportive and inclusive environment. The strengths-based approach has proven effective in achieving specific workplace outcomes, demonstrating that this method empowers both leaders and staff, enhancing their sense of competence and confidence in their abilities [267]. This method aligns with feeling psychologically safe in the workplace, which we will discuss in chapter 7.

DYSLEXIA

Will right brainers rule the world, asked Daniel Pink? Daniel Pink, the author of *A Whole New Mind: Why right-brainers Will Rule the Future* is a fascinating insight into our thinking, almost two decades ago. Pink's book explores that changing working environments and the impact of advancing technologies, artificial intelligence (AI) and a transient global workforce - if only he could have seen what COVID would do! Fast forward to 2024, and we are watching the rapid advances in technology, a global workforce where offshoring has become the new way to work, and we can now work anywhere from the comfort of our own home. Additionally, AI is moving so rapidly that humans can't keep up … hello ChatGPT!

So, what does this have to do with Pink's book? He hypothesised that those who work in traditional job roles and use more of their left brain, such as finance and manufacturing, could be replaced by AI. And he wasn't wrong. We are seeing a huge shift in the types of job roles currently being affected by AI. Ernst and Young found that previous workforce augmentation, which involves automating certain aspects of jobs to complement and enhance the human workforce, has traditionally been a secondary consideration in CEOs' strategic initiatives. However, it is now emerging as a key driver of organisational efficiency. Software-based automation, including Robotic Process Automation and Intelligent Process Automation (encompassing Machine Learning, Deep Learning, Natural Language Processing, and Chatbots), is significantly transforming our workplaces at an extraordinary pace, and we will need to collaborate between human and automated efforts as automation continues to grow [266]. We will talk further about how dyslexics are collaborating with AI to get their jobs done. The direct impact of automation on the workforce will lead to a notable transformation in the skills and capabilities required to adapt to the evolving demands of human roles [266].

SHAE WISSEL

I'm rambling, so let's get to the point. Dyslexics are typically right-brain dominant compared to non-dyslexics. Personal resources and soft skills seem to play a crucial role in work engagement and how dyslexic employees navigate and adapt to the working environment. These skills are going to become more valuable in the workplace because they cannot be replaced by AI, yet. Let's look at what this might mean for your workplace.

Personal resources are defined as individual attributes that are often associated with resilience, providing individuals with a sense of control and the ability to effectively navigate their environment [268]. Researchers examined possible factors that could contribute to the success of people with dyslexia, including, perseverance, resilience, initiative, lateral thinking, idea generation and reasoning abilities, self-awareness, empathy coping strategies visual-spatial thinking, creativity, complex problem-solving ability, innovative, big-picture strategic thinking and establishing creating support systems [266, 269, 270]. People with dyslexia who were able to develop intuitive personal strategies to manage workplace stresses, were also more likely to experience a successful working environment and career [163, 269].

Figure 10 Dyslexic strengths from participant from my research.

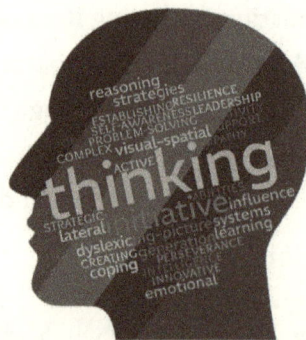

Although dyslexics are consistently exposed to stressful difficulties that they must overcome, my research found that dyslexics appear to do this by drawing on their personal resources to manage and succeed in the workplace. Examples include resilience, perseverance, building human connections, empathy, creative and strategic thinking, agility of thought and exceptional leadership skills (See Figure.10). Those who could employ these traits seemed to do better in life overall, which is in line with other research showing that with successful adaptation, dyslexics can have overall improved quality of life [97, 271].

As we move into an age of automation and artificial intelligence, these strengths can be a powerful tool in unlocking new opportunities and driving innovation. Sir Richard Branson and Made By Dyslexia launched *The Intelligence 5.0, a new school of thought rethinking the intelligence needed in the Industry 5* report[272]. Literally, as I was finalising my book, when the report was launched In the report listed six *Dyslexic Thinking skills*: visualising, imagining, communicating, reasoning, connecting, and exploring were discussed. This links back to the discussion earlier about the concept of Dyslexic Thinking. The report states that these skills will become invaluable as we move into the AI era, where humans will need to collaborate with AI tools , so watch this space. While there may be individual differences in the extent to which these skills are developed, it's encouraging to hear that our research demonstrated high levels of self-efficacy and resilience among individuals with dyslexia. By recognising and leveraging these strengths, individuals with dyslexia can thrive in a variety of different roles and industries. By actively recruiting dyslexics into businesses and tapping into their talents such as leadership and social influence, creativity, originality and initiative ensures diverse workforces that can be remain relevant into the future.

4.8. CONCLUSION

This was a big chapter, they all are. By working through this chapter, you will now know that the challenges encountered by dyslexics in the workplace are more than just difficulties in areas such as reading but are much broader, impacting on executive functioning skills, written expression and maths, and we haven't even touched on mental health in the workplace yet. These difficulties, shaped by the various characteristics of dyslexia, emphasise the need for individualised support so dyslexics can thrive in the workplace enabling them to work to their full potential. When support is in place, it enables those with dyslexia to work to their strengths, and this can lead to high-performing teams. In the rapidly changing work environment, driven by AI, we will see the need for the personal resources and skills of dyslexic employees; recognising and harnessing these skills will contribute to sustainable and innovative practices in the future.

KEY TAKE-HOME MESSAGES

Holistic Support Approach: Understanding dyslexia as a spectrum is crucial for providing holistic support, recognising that challenges vary across the employment life cycle.

Strength-Based Perspective: Embracing a strength-based approach is essential, highlighting and leveraging the unique strengths dyslexic individuals bring, including creative thinking, resilience, and problem-solving skills.

Individualised Support Strategies: Recognising that dyslexia affects individuals differently emphasises the need for tailored support strategies that address specific challenges throughout one's career.

Positive Work Environments: Creating a positive and inclusive work environment involves acknowledging dyslexia as a spectrum and appreciating the strengths dyslexic individuals contribute to the workplace.

Change is coming: As we navigate an era of automation and artificial intelligence, the identified strengths of dyslexic individuals become valuable assets, driving innovation and the soft skills needed that, at the moment, AI can't replace.

Continuous Learning and Adaptation: To build and retain a strong workforce inclusive of dyslexic individuals, continuous learning, reflection and implementation of support measures are essential for adapting to the evolving nature of work.

Celebrating Diversity of strengths, perspectives, and approaches is key to thriving in the workplace, and dyslexic individuals contribute significantly to this diversity.

Individual Growth and Well-being: Encouraging self-advocacy, personal growth and well-being among dyslexic individuals, involves recognising and building upon their strengths rather than focusing solely on overcoming challenges.

These take-home messages emphasise the importance of embracing diversity, fostering inclusivity and leveraging the unique strengths of dyslexic individuals for personal and collective success in the workplace.

Chapter 5
DO YOU SEE ME, TO DISCLOSE OR NOT TO DISCLOSE

Anything is possible when you have the right people there to support you.
Misty Copeland, African American Ballet Dancer

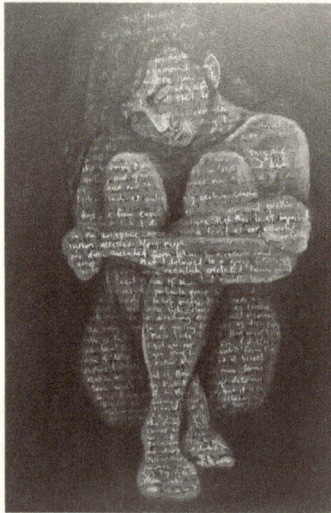

5.1. TO DISCLOSE OR NOT TO DISCLOSE - THAT IS THE QUESTION.

'...No, I kept it [dyslexia] very much a secret. I saw so much judgment and prejudice about dyslexic people that, given the jobs I did, at the very centre of them was being clever. I wasn't going to create prejudice around it towards me, so I never shared that...'

Research participant

One of the most important and personal decisions that individuals with disabilities, such as dyslexia, face is whether to disclose their condition. We have identified through my research and work three distinct types of personas in the workplace regarding dyslexic employees as illustrated in Figure.11.

Image 11. The three persona's in the workpalce

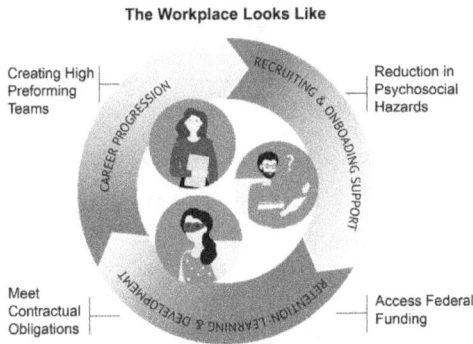

The Workplace Looks Like

Creating High Preforming Teams

Reduction in Psychosocial Hazards

Meet Contractual Obligations

Access Federal Funding

The first type is individuals, like me, who are open about their dyslexia. This openness often stems, for some, from a fear of being discovered while concealing this aspect of their identity, which can hinder their ability to present their true selves in the workplace. While some individuals in this category are willing to discuss their experiences, they may not wish to serve as representatives for the dyslexic community, in or out of the workplace, or participate in disability working groups. They have developed their own strategies for managing their dyslexia or have workplace accommodations in place, and prefer to focus on their job responsibilities. Those in this category tend to be in high-profile positions who, with many happy to share that they have dyslexia but do not want to be a poster person for it or to lead any workplace reforms.

The second type consists of individuals who are concealing their dyslexia, choosing not to disclose their condition. This cohort is struggling in silence and needs your help.

The third type includes individuals who are struggling in the workplace but are uncertain about the reasons behind their challenges. They might exhibit various dyslexic traits, without having had the opportunity for assessment. It is often only through the assessment of a child or family member, that they realise they may also be dyslexic. Many of these individuals have not encountered the concept of dyslexia before and may hold a poor self-concept, believing they are unintelligent or slower than their peers. This negative self-perception may have been reinforced by ongoing external feedback throughout their lives, leading to issues around self-concept, self-worth and self-belief. So, let's break this down as to why someone may not disclose in the workplace.

Disability researchers indicate that revealing one's disability in the workplace can lead to negative repercussions across various facets of a worker's life, including physical and mental health, social relationships and job performance. As mentioned earlier, the decision to share one's dyslexia is complicated, making it a difficult choice in most cases [273-275]. As highlighted earlier, the research tells us that many feel they will be disadvantaged if they disclose their dyslexia, which can contribute to their reluctance to identify their 'disability' [276]. I want to reinforce these facts here again. In the workplace, individuals may encounter several challenges that hinder them from disclosing their dyslexia. These challenges include perceptions of potential discrimination and stigmatisation, the prevailing workplace culture, such as the availability of reasonable adjustments to support their roles post-disclosure, limited awareness and understanding, workplace dynamics (whether supportive or high-pressure), concerns regarding the impact of disclosure on career advancement and lack of psychological-safety [274, 277, 278]. Beetham and Okhai (2017) identified that individuals often hesitate to disclose their dyslexia due to fears of possible victimisation by their employer or bullying from colleagues.

My research found that dyslexics were more likely to disclose to people close to them, including friends and family, rather than to people at work (90% v. 57%) [98]. This supports the work of Alexander-Passe (2015) who found that individuals are only inclined to disclose their learning disability if they feel comfortable or well-supported. We also found that dyslexics were too fearful to disclose their difficulties in at least one job and would mask, pass or conceal their difficulties instead. Others indicated they felt forced to disclose their dyslexia if they felt threatened (for example, if their performance was being questioned) [256]. Disclosure in this scenario is unlikely to produce a positive outcome, as the dyslexic employee feels like they have been backed into a corner.

However, it's not all bad. Other studies have reported that voluntary disclosure of a disability can led to positive outcomes and has been shown to alleviate the stress of concealing an invisible disability [139, 279]. It may reduce feelings of isolation by enabling individuals to establish social connections with supportive individuals and to request workplace accommodations that enable improved job performance [160, 279].

5.2. HOW TO DISCLOSE MY DYSLEXIA TO MY MANAGER AND OR EMPLOYER

This next section has been developed to support those who want to disclose and those who may think their team member/employee may be dyslexic. These are based on my personal experiences, and you should seek professional advice and support as well. I'm including this because I'm often asked by those that have dyslexia or those who work with people who they think are dyslexic, what the best way is to broach the topic. Below are some suggestions and thoughts I've had over the years on how we can do this in a positive, supportive way.

I frequently engage with individuals with dyslexia who are considering disclosing their condition to their managers. There are several reasons for this desire for disclosure; some wish to be their true, authentic selves in the workplace, while others feel that the timing is right for them. Many seek guidance on when the appropriate time for disclosure might be. As previously mentioned, this decision is highly personal and varies from individual to individual. I usually wait until after my probationary period of employment, because that's when I feel the safest to talk about my difficulties, and I know that I'm protected under the Discrimination Act and the Fair Work Act. When you're in a probationary period, an employer can terminate your contract and there's nothing you can do about it. I was once terminated in a probationary period because of my dyslexia difficulties, and it was devastating. The power imbalance and its effect on your self-esteem are significant, and no one wants to feel like that in a job. When an individual approaches me for guidance on disclosing their dyslexia, I recommend they do so with a sense of empowerment and a readiness to educate their employer or manager. It is essential to recognise that many managers or employers lack training and awareness regarding dyslexia and the implications of having a hidden disability. Below are some suggested steps to consider:

Self-Reflection: Before disclosing, reflect on how dyslexia affects your job role and whether disclosing would benefit you. What is the purpose of disclosing? Is it to access support, like workplace accommodations, to raise awareness in your workplace, to feel more confident? Consider the specific challenges you face and potential accommodations you require to support you in your job role.

Understanding Your Rights: Familiarise yourself with the company's policies regarding disability disclosure and accommodations. Understand your rights under relevant laws, such as the Disability Discrimination ACT 1992 and the Fair Work Act 2010 or its equivalent in your region. You could also speak with the Australian Human Rights Commission for support on knowing your rights around workplace accommodations.

You can look on the Fair Work Ombudsman website: https://www.fairwork.gov.au/ . They will provide you with tailored advice and information. Further details are in the resource section.

Understand your workplace: Review your organisation's policies and procedures. Do they have a disclosure policy? What accommodations can you access that might be helpful, such as flexitime, working from home, and tools that are already available? Be prepared and knowledgeable about your workplace rights.

Does your workplace have an Ability Committee? Check if your organisation has an Ability committee or DEI committee that you can speak with. Do they help to advocate for your needs? What is their role, and how can they help?

Talk with HR: If you haven't already, initiate a conversation with your HR team and/or DEI team if you have one. Seek their support and advice on how to approach discussing dyslexia with your manager. They can provide valuable insights and guidance.

Schedule a Meeting: Arrange a meeting with your manager and HR to discuss your dyslexia. If you feel the need bring a support person along, maybe someone from DEI or from an Ability or other committee that would help be a second pair of ears for you. Having both parties present ensures a comprehensive understanding and facilitates a collaborative approach.

Prepare Resources: Assume that your manager may not have an in-depth understanding of dyslexia. Gather resources such as our factsheets, online materials and the Dear Dyslexic podcasts available on **re:think dyslexia**. These resources can serve as educational tools for your manager.

Highlight Your Strengths: During the meeting, emphasise the strengths of your role. Discuss how dyslexia has shaped your unique skillset and contributions to the team.

Requesting accommodations: Clearly articulate the support you need to perform at your best, whether it's specific technologies, quiet time, flexibility to work from home or learning and development support from a dyslexia specialist. Take any tools that are already helping you or could help you, such as Grammarly.

Set a Follow-up Meeting: Conclude the initial discussion by setting a follow-up meeting. This session can explore specific ways your manager can support you in your role. It provides an opportunity to address any additional questions or concerns they may have and what accommodations you can access.

Key Tips:

- **Be Open and Honest:** Approach the conversation with openness and honesty. Share your experiences and challenges candidly to foster understanding.

- **Educate Gently:** Use the gathered resources to educate your manager about dyslexia gently. Offer insights into how they can support you effectively.
- **Focus on Solutions:** Frame the conversation positively by focusing on solutions and the types of support that you need to perform best in your job role.
- **Encourage Questions:** Ask HR to help create an environment where everyone feels comfortable to asking questions. Address any misconceptions and provide clarity on how dyslexia impacts your work.

By following this guide, you hopefully, feel empowered to have a productive and open conversation about dyslexia and your needs with your manager and HR, fostering a workplace that values diversity and inclusivity. This way, you're self-advocating for your needs and also able to talk about what you do well on the job and, most importantly, educate them. I know this shouldn't be our job, and hopefully, in time, this will change.

Also, it is important to identify the tools and resources available to enable you to do your job to the best of your ability. Outlining a list of these tools and resources again helps to educate and empower your manager to provide you with the resources you need. You can find further information on workplace accommodations and support, including JobAccess in Chapter 8: Setting Dyslexic Talent Up for Success in the Workplace. If you are unsure what tools can help, then call **1800 13 NEAP (6327)** to find out more.

5.3. HOW TO TALK TO A TEAM MEMBER WHO YOU THINK MIGHT BE DYSLEXIC

'What do you do if you think a team member might be dyslexic?' I get asked

this question quite often, particularly when I'm doing presentations or running training sessions. A manager or team member has seen a team member have reading and writing difficulties, and they are unsure how to broach the topic with them. This is an important question and one with no straightforward answer, because everybody is different, and the way they respond in the situation depends on the trauma and baggage they might be carrying. The only reason I found out I was dyslexic, was because my tutor at the time sat me down and told me that *she thought I was dyslexic*. If she hadn't said that, I would have been roaming the world thinking I was dumb, stupid and slow! So, I am forever grateful to my tutor, Lisa, who had the foresight and the ability to have that brave conversation with me. Now, consequent to this, I might have had my first, and hopefully only ever, mental health crisis, but these words changed my life and you could change someone else's as well. Having those brave conversations in the workplace can be really challenging, especially when you're worried how it might be perceived by the other person. As difficult as it is, you need to do what is right for the employee and your organisation. Here are my suggested strategies:

Guide: Navigating a Supportive Conversation about Dyslexia in the Workplace

Supporting team members with dyslexia involves open communication and understanding. Here's a guide on how to have a constructive conversation with your Human Resources team, or manager, about addressing difficulties that a team member may be facing. It is important to look at what your policies and procedures state about supporting neurodivergent employees and use these as a guide.

Starting the conversation: Initiate a conversation with your HR and or P&C team and/or manager to discuss what you have observed and the difficulties that the team member is demonstrating; you need to create examples so you can help them.

Educate Yourself: Prior to the conversation, educate yourself about dyslexia and the available resources. This will equip you to approach the discussion with a well-informed perspective. Find out what is already available in your workplace. What do your policies and procedures say? What tools are already available? If you need more information look at rethinkdyslexia.com.au

Start with Strengths: Begin the conversation by acknowledging and emphasising the positive aspects of the team member's performance. Highlight their strengths and contributions to set a positive tone.

Outline Concerns with Evidence: Present documented evidence of the difficulties you've observed, framing it as a mismatch in abilities, where strengths and challenges coexist. Use language that is neutral and objective to avoid judgment. You don't have to directly say, '*are you dyslexic?*'

Give Time for Processing: Allow the team member time to process the information and encourage them to ask questions. They might choose to disclose their dyslexia or share personal experiences related to their challenges, or they may not, and that's ok as well. Give them time to go away and think about the conversation.

Offer Support: Provide support for areas where they are struggling. Offer tools for improving grammar and spelling, inquire about the need for extra time to complete tasks, discuss flexible working arrangements, suggest more regular breaks, or provide access to a quiet workspace. Mention available mental health support such as our 1800 13 NEAP (6327) Neurodivergent Employment Assistance Program, or you might have an Employee Assistance Program in place.

Approach with Empathy: Come to the conversation with empathy, ensuring it is a collaborative dialogue rather than a confrontational one. Present options and solutions to make it a supportive and empowering discussion. Link them in with other programs in your workplace as well as EAP support if you have it.

Explore Dyslexia Services: If they express interest in understanding their challenges better, recommend resources like **re:think dyslexia** for a private consultation. We offer dyslexia screening and other services to provide valuable insights.

Plan for a Follow-up: Conclude the initial meeting with a plan for a follow-up session. Outline the next steps to be taken, including any adjustments to be made, additional support provided, or further discussions that may be necessary.

Consistent feedback is essential for all employee development. Establish a feedback loop that includes regular check-ins to provide constructive insights into performance and where they are improving. Give them time to adjust to any new tools or strategies they implement. Learning new tools and creating new habits all take time, and extra time is what is needed. This is not a *one-size-fits*-all approach to supporting dyslexia and other neurodivergent employees; everyone is different, and it takes time to work through what tools and accommodations work. It is important to highlight both strengths and areas for improvement, creating an environment where the employee feels comfortable asking questions and seeking clarification. Working from a strength-based approach is important for the whole team, not just those who are dyslexic. Maintaining a routine of consistent feedback, enabling workplace accommodations that meet the needs of the individual, and upskilling yourself as the manager can reduce the need for challenging conversations and performance management plans. Laying the foundation of trust and psychological safety for the whole team. If in doubt call **re:think dyslexia** on 1800 13 63 27.

5.4. CONCLUSION

This chapter discussed the three distinct dyslexic personas in the workplace. Firstly, there are individuals like me who openly disclose their difficulties. This open disclosure may be due to several reasons, such as a fear of being exposed and a desire to bring their true, authentic selves to the workplace. Alternatively, they may feel comfortable in their current role and do not believe disclosing will jeopardise their career. These individuals may not necessarily want to be spokespersons for dyslexia but are willing to discuss it while maintaining their strategies for success. Secondly, some struggle in silence due to a lack of awareness or opportunity for assessment and are unsure why. Lastly, some individuals mask, pass and or conceal their dyslexia due to fear of discrimination and the potential negative impact this could have on their employment and career opportunities.

The decision to disclose dyslexia in the workplace is complex and influenced by various factors, as discussed. Concerns about workplace discrimination, stigmatisation, workplace culture, relationships, and the perceived impact on career progression are all significant obstacles to disclosure. Individuals with dyslexia may fear victimisation or bullying if they choose to disclose, highlighting the need for a supportive work environment.

The last section provides practical guidance for those considering disclosure and those aiming to support team members with dyslexia. It emphasises the importance of empowerment, self-advocacy, and creating a safe space for conversations. For disclosing to managers or employers, steps include involving HR, setting up a meeting, providing resources and highlighting strengths and support needs.

When approaching a team member whom you suspect might be dyslexic, the suggestions include initiating a conversation with HR or management, educating yourself about dyslexia, focusing on strengths, documenting observed difficulties, offering support options and ensuring follow-up meetings for further steps.

In essence, developing an open and supportive workplace culture, backed by education and understanding, and easy access to workplace accommodation, is essential for addressing the challenges associated with disclosing dyslexia. Encouraging brave conversations and providing appropriate support can contribute to creating an inclusive and accommodating work environment for individuals with dyslexia - and everyone can thrive!

KEY TAKE-HOME MESSAGES

Diverse Workplace Personas: There are three distinct personas regarding dyslexia disclosure in the workplace. Individuals openly disclosing may vary in their willingness to be advocates or label themselves, while others choose to mask their condition. Some struggle silently, often lacking awareness or assessment opportunities.

Complex Decision-Making: The decision to disclose dyslexia is multifaceted and deeply personal. Fear of discrimination, workplace culture, relationships and concerns about career progression act as significant barriers to disclosure. Creating a psychologically safe supportive work environment is crucial for overcoming these obstacles.

Selective Disclosure: Individuals with dyslexia are more likely to disclose to friends and family than to colleagues. Fear of repercussions or feeling compelled to disclose under duress, are common reasons for not sharing in certain job situations. The workplace should strive to be a space where disclosure is met with understanding and support.

Support Strategies for Disclosure: For those considering disclosure, empowerment and self-advocacy are crucial. Practical steps include involving HR, setting up informed meetings with managers, providing resources, highlighting strengths and outlining support needs.

Building awareness and understanding within the workplace is vital.

Initiating Brave Conversations: Recognising dyslexia in team members requires empathy and careful consideration. Initiating conversations with HR, educating oneself about dyslexia, focusing on strengths, documenting difficulties and offering support options are essential strategies. Follow-up meetings ensure ongoing support.

Creating an Inclusive Culture: Fostering an open and supportive workplace culture is key to addressing challenges related to dyslexia disclosure. Encouraging brave conversations and providing support can contribute to building a psychologically safe environment where individuals with dyslexia feel valued and empowered.

The workplace plays a crucial role in supporting individuals with dyslexia. Understanding the diverse perspectives and challenges surrounding disclosure, fostering a culture of empathy and support, psychological safety and implementing practical strategies, are essential for creating an inclusive and accommodating work environment for everyone.

DISCLOSURE FRAMEWORK FOR THE WORKPLACE

Purpose: This framework is designed to encourage open communication and voluntary disclosure/sharing of dyslexia by employees within your workplace. The goal is to create an inclusive and supportive environment for all employees, ensuring that individuals with dyslexia have the resources and accommodations they need to excel in their roles.

Voluntary Disclosure:

Voluntary Nature: Disclosure of dyslexia is entirely voluntary. Employees are encouraged to share information about their dyslexia only if they feel comfortable and believe it is necessary for their work.

Confidentiality: Any information disclosed will be treated with the utmost confidentiality. Only relevant personnel directly involved in providing support and accommodations will be informed, ensuring privacy for the disclosing individual.

Process:

Initiating Disclosure:

- Employees may choose to disclose their dyslexia to their immediate supervisor or the designated HR representative.
- Disclosures can be made verbally or in writing, depending on the employee's preference.

Information Shared:

- Employees disclosing dyslexia may provide information about the specific challenges they face and any accommodations or adjustments they believe would be beneficial.

Needs Assessment:

- Upon disclosure, HR or designated personnel will work with the employee to assess their needs, considering both job-specific requirements and general workplace support.

Accommodations and Support:

Individualised Accommodations:

- Reasonable accommodations will be provided based on the needs identified during the disclosure process. This may include assistive technologies, flexible work arrangements, or modified communication methods and access to coaching and 1:1 support.

Training and Awareness:

- The workplace will conduct training sessions to increase awareness about dyslexia, reducing stigma and fostering a more inclusive environment for all employees.

Ongoing Communication:
Review and Feedback:

Employees and relevant personnel will have periodic reviews to assess the effectiveness of accommodations and make adjustments as needed.

Continuous Support:

- The workplace will maintain an open-door policy for ongoing communication, ensuring that employees feel supported in discussing their needs and challenges related to dyslexia.

Non-Discrimination Assurance:

Equal Opportunities: Disclosure of dyslexia will not affect an employee's opportunities for advancement, promotion or any other aspects of their career within the organisation.

By implementing this Dyslexia Disclosure Framework, your workplace aims to create an environment where employees feel comfortable, supported, and empowered to perform at their best.

RESOURCES

There are a huge number of resources you can find, so we are listing just a few to help you on your journey of discovery and understanding. You can find more information at

- rethink dyslexia.com.au. If you found any of this content distressing, please seek support:
- Lifeline on 13 11 14
- BeyondBlue counsellor on 1300 22 4636 NEAP Neurodivergent Employment Assistance Program on 1800 13 6327

Helplines:

- Australian Human Rights Commission website: https://humanrights.gov.au/. Or phone number: 1300 369 711. Hours are 9:00 AM - 5:00 PM AEST/AEDT.

Fair Work Ombudsman website: https://www.fairwork.gov.au/ or call 13 13 94 between 8:00 am – 5:30 pm Monday to Friday to speak with an adviser. They will provide you with tailored advice and information

- Peer support
- Dear Dyslexic closed Adult Facebook group
- Dear Dyslexic PhD and dyslexic researcher

Chapter 6
UNRAVELLING WORKPLACE CHALLENGES: RECOGNISING INTERNAL BARRIERS

'...I hold three degrees: a Bachelor of Arts with Honours, a Master of Cultural and Communication Studies from the University of Sydney, and a Master of Cultural Studies and a Bachelor of Arts from the University of Tasmania. My academic background includes theatre, cultural studies, and communication, and I have a specialisation in performance studies. Additionally, I engage in volunteer work with Fellow Travellers who are neurodiverse. Over the past nine years, I have undertaken eight overseas trips supported by scholarships and fellowships, the most recent of which was the Churchill Fellowship, aimed at concluding my research on neurodiversity in the performing arts in the United States and the United Kingdom.

Despite these qualifications and experiences, I can't get a job.

I am often perceived as "normal," albeit hyperactive, and I have been
informed that I possess an exceptional memory…'
Dan, a dyslexic community member

This chapter looks at dyslexia across the employment life cycle for transitioning into the workforce through career progression. Gainful employment goes far beyond financial security and economic independence. Being employed enables social interactions, supports positive mental health and allows individuals to participate meaningfully in society [280]. Long-term unemployment and underemployment can have adverse effects on mental health and well-being and lead to financial strain and social isolation [280, 281]. While various factors can contribute to employment challenges, individuals with disabilities often experience higher unemployment rates compared to their counterparts without disabilities [241, 243]. In the Australian workforce, working-age individuals with disabilities, including those with dyslexia, constitute 53%, contrasting with 84% among those without disabilities. The unemployment rate for individuals with disabilities (8.3%) tends to be higher than that for those without disabilities (5.3%), depending on the year of publication [241, 242].

Local and international research has found that, despite difficulties, most individuals with dyslexia enter the labour market after completing their secondary or tertiary education [31, 98, 212, 282]. Yet, there is limited evidence in Australia examining how educational attainment can affect employment outcomes for individuals with dyslexia. An international study by Dubow et al. (2006) found there was a considerable association between children's cognitive/academic functioning at age eight (measured by an IQ test in one study and teacher ratings of school achievement in another study) and occupational outcomes at 42 and 48 years of age. Other studies [283, 284] have shown that reading problems can lead to early school departure, resulting in low levels of formal educational qualifications and limited occupational choices. A study based in the Isle of Wight in the UK also found an 'understandable reluctance [of people with dyslexia] to consider entering jobs with high literacy demands and this meant that most went into unskilled or manual occupations as they left school, and many remained in manual roles later in their lives' [283]. International and my local research demonstrates that dyslexics are employed across various sectors and industries, with a cross-section of unskilled roles through to middle management, senior management, executive level and board roles [98, 110, 212, 269, 284, 285]. My research found that 38% of dyslexics were working at levels lower than they were qualified for, [98] a finding backed by the international literature [211, 287]. This combined research suggests that career progression may be more difficult for working dyslexics, which we will explore in section 6.5: Career progression.

To start, let's look at what life is like for young people as they transition out of education into the workforce. We will then look at the types of barriers facing dyslexics across the employment life cycle, from recruitment to career progression. I hope you take some key insight away from this section and what can be done to improve employment opportunities for those with dyslexia.

6.1. TRANSITIONING INTO THE WORKPLACE FROM SCHOOL - HOW WE CAN SUPPORT YOUNG ADULTS.

Transitioning into the workplace can be stressful for anyone, let alone someone who is dyslexic. For most young people, they will have had a part-time job while at school or university. Commencing formal employment is often a scary and exciting time. No research yet looks at young dyslexics as they transition into adulthood and the workplace. However, there is research that indicates that young individuals who are neither enrolled in education, training, nor engaged in paid employment by the age of 24 face an elevated risk of enduring prolonged unemployment in the future [286]. Statistics reveal that one in three Australians aged 24, particularly those from the lowest socio-economic backgrounds, are not participating in education, employment or training [286]. We know that young people with dyslexia are at risk of disengaging in education and may find it difficult to be employed [287]. To reduce this risk, early intervention during the school years is vital in supporting young people to finish secondary school and have the opportunity to enter TAFE, higher education or go straight into the workforce. Proactively equipping young people with the skills and tools before they enter adulthood will reduce the risk of obtaining meaningful employment and increase their opportunities for a successful future in the workforce.

I want to take you down memory lane and share a personal story before we look at what's happening in Australia for our young people and those completing higher education.

I was over the moon with happiness when I was employed in my first formal job as a graduate speech pathologist, way back when. I was so proud of myself even though I had struggled significantly at university. I had been laughed at and told, at one point, I wouldn't be able to graduate due to my poor writing skills. Even so, the thrill of being employed at a rehabilitation hospital was wonderful; only a handful of graduates received a job like this. For the first time in a long time, I didn't feel dumb!

As I embarked on my first year after graduating, I was filled with enthusiasm and a strong sense of purpose. I believed I was destined to excel as a speech pathologist. Initially, I was eager and committed, enthusiastically moving through hospital wards and engaging with my patients. However, it wasn't long before I encountered challenges that shook my confidence. I struggled with certain aspects of my job, such as correctly pronouncing and spelling words. I found myself getting confused about the regions of the brain associated with language processing, like Wernicke and Broca. Questions like, 'Where are they located?' and 'How do you spell them again?' constantly plagued my mind.

Despite my genuine connection with patients, my difficulties became glaringly evident when completing handwritten medical records. My notes were riddled with spelling and grammatical errors, and poor handwriting soon became a source of increasing frustration for my manager. She didn't hold back her dissatisfaction, often berating me in front of colleagues and openly expressing regret for hiring me. Her disdain was palpable, making me feel inadequate and constantly on edge.

I spent long hours at work, staying late every night to try and meticulously write my notes while striving to avoid errors and the scrutiny of others. Keeping up with the required reading was another struggle. Journal articles presented a daunting challenge, filled with complex terminology and unfamiliar numbers. I dreaded the prospect of delivering these articles during professional team development sessions, fearing I wouldn't grasp the content or be able to convey it effectively. My anxiety reached its peak when I faced the prospect of speaking in front of the entire medical team during our fortnightly multidisciplinary team meetings. The fear of stumbling over words or failing to explain concepts correctly, loomed large, leading me to worry incessantly about being perceived as incompetent. This introduction into my first professional role was horrible; no wonder I was suicidal after being diagnosed with dyslexia and dysgraphia. The trauma I carried was significant. What young people experience in their first professional job can leave an indelible impression and we want young people, no matter what industry they are in, to be set up for success, not for failure as I experienced. Setting dyslexic young people up for success in their first professional job out of school or university involves a combination of preparation, support and understanding. Many of the tools and recommendations are relevant to any employee with dyslexia, but I think there are a few key things to consider when we enter our first role, regardless of the industry.

The reason Im sharing this is to help you understand the complexities for a young person but also what we are currently seeing for those who are completing higher education and what the trajectory looks like for some dyslexic graduates. Their story could be my story if I was finishing my degree. The research tells us that many young Australians with dyslexia are going to TAFE and university, as mentioned earlier. A high proportion of dyslexics are completing their bachelor's degree. Yet we have learnt that some dyslexics who have completed their university degrees in education and health struggle to pass the literacy and numeracy tests required to finalise their degree. For teaching, this is the Literacy and Numeracy Test for Initial Teacher Education Students. In health, these may be the literacy and numeracy tests administered by the Australian Health Practitioner Regulation Agency. Such tests pose significant challenges to successfully completing them without appropriate accommodations. When accommodations are provided, they often lack the necessary customisation to meet dyslexics. As a result, many students face significant obstacles in finalising their degrees, which can lead to financial strain due to years of investment in their education without the opportunity to enter their chosen professions.

This situation creates a cycle of disadvantage, as individuals may incur substantial debt and either need to retrain or work in roles that do not align with their qualifications, which raises concerns of discrimination. While some may argue that those who cannot complete these assessments are unsuitable for teaching or healthcare roles, it is crucial to recognise that they are placed at an unfair disadvantage without access to the appropriate support tools.

Governments are crying out for more educators and healthcare professionals; Australia is in a healthcare and education crisis now. Not enough workers, people are leaving these professions in droves and yet the existing regulations do not provide dyslexic individuals with an equitable opportunity to complete their degrees. I believe that if I had a dyslexic teacher during my education, someone who could provide empathy, patience and understanding, I would have felt less fearful and ashamed and more supported throughout my educational journey. It is imperative that governments and regulatory bodies consider these perspectives in their policies and practices so that those with dyslexia are not unfairly disadvantaged financially and in their ability to work in their chosen professions. I know if I was completing a bachelor's in speech pathology now or education, I would not be able to qualify because of these tests, and yet I have four degrees! So, as a fellow dyslexic, it's extremely concerning that this is happening to those in the dyslexic community and to many others where English might be the second language, for example.

Ok, now that we have looked at a significant barrier for some graduates, let's look at what can happen to young people when they are employed in their first formal job and how we can set them up to succeed, unlike my story!

One of the first barriers they may encounter is the lack of workplace accommodations that they readily receive at school, TAFE or university if they were diagnosed during their schooling years. These young people may have received accommodations, such as extra time for assignments and exams, and access to different types of technology, such as text-to-speech and speech-to-text. So, when they enter the workforce, they will expect this type of support, and it is often a shock when they find these are not easily accessible. What might have been open dialogue at school now becomes a topic that can't be discussed, and their difficulties are unable to be shared because they don't feel safe to do so, as discussed earlier. They may struggle without the accommodations they were able to access at school, TAFE or university, and now they are floundering. Or perhaps they are like me when they graduate and enter the workforce, without even knowing that they have these types of difficulties, so they continue to make mistakes that start as an annoyance, become a frustration and then a performance management issue. And this is what we want to see.

Supporting a young person in a new job role is essential for their professional growth and success. To help them adjust and thrive in their new position, it's important to take several key strategies into consideration that you, as a parent, secondary schools, TAFE, University, and workplace, can do to support a smooth transition into formal employment. As you read through or listen, reflect on what you feel your education setting or workplace is currently doing well and where there could be areas for improvement.

Building Self-Advocacy and Independence: Starting at Home

It's essential to begin developing self-advocacy skills at home, empowering young people to take control of their own needs and aspirations. By parents, family and educators encourage them to take the lead in what will happen for them once they leave school. This could look like supporting them to complete paperwork for TAFE or Uni, helping them creating their CV and employment documents. While it's tempting to step in and do these activities for them, it's more beneficial to guide them through the process, providing support where needed. Tools like ChatGPT can be invaluable in helping them articulate their thoughts and structure their documents effectively. However, the key is to let them do the work, offering feedback and assistance without taking over.

This process is about more than just paperwork; it's about promoting independence. In the workplace, they won't have someone by their side to handle tasks for them. Learning to navigate and build these skills independently will equip them with the confidence and tools they'll need as they transition into adulthood.

Practicing Social Skills and Building Connections

Beyond technical skills, social skills are crucial for success in and out of the workplace. Encourage young people to practice interacting with a variety of people, particularly adults, to build comfort and confidence in different types of settings. This could involve role-playing scenarios at home or arranging for them to spend time with a mentor - someone who can offer insights, guidance and support as they prepare to enter the workforce and become more independent. Mentorship with an adult with dyslexia and/or other neurodivergence, can be particularly valuable, providing young people with a role model who understands the challenges they face and to draw on their strengths and can help them navigate the complexities of workplace dynamics.

Promoting Autonomy and Self-Determination in Secondary School

As young people move through secondary school, it's important to encourage the use of tools and strategies that support their learning and organisation. This might include using technology to assist with reading and writing and developing systems to stay on top of assignments and deadlines. The goal is to help them build autonomy and self-determination, skills that are critical for success in both higher education and the workplace.

Building resilience and confidence is equally important. The transition to adulthood and the workforce is an exciting time and, at times, can be challenging with or without being neurodivergent. Young people will need to be prepared to face setbacks and persevere. Encouraging a growth mindset, where they see challenges as opportunities to learn and grow, can help them build the resilience they need.

Teach them conflict resolution skills and provide guidance on how to handle conflicts is essential for managing in the workplace. Make sure they are aware of the appropriate channels for reporting issues. Encourage them to build professional relationships within the organisation through networking. This can help them learn from others, seek mentorship and advance in their careers. This could include accessing and/or participating in your disability and/or neurodivergent network. Empower them to take initiative and make decisions within their scope of responsibility.

Supporting Neurodivergent Individuals in the Workplace

Once young people enter the workforce, workplaces must be equipped to support neurodivergent individuals, from recruitment through to career progression. This support should include accommodations and resources tailored to their unique needs and a culture that values diversity and inclusivity. This chapter will discuss these aspects further, highlighting the importance of creating a workplace environment where neurodivergent individuals can thrive.

Encourage a flexible approach to work arrangements, when possible, to accommodate their needs. Provide access to employee assistance programs or resources that support their mental and emotional well-being. Remember that each young person is unique, so tailor your support strategies to their needs and preferences. Regular communication and a genuine interest in their professional growth will go a long way in helping them succeed in their new job role. For additional tips and ideas, listen to the Dear Dyslexic Podcast on supporting neurodivergent young people in the workplace with Deidre Hardy.

6.2. RECRUITMENT AND ONBOARDING PRACTICES

'...I did not make public my disability; in fact, I remember the form I had to sign to gain employment, which said, "Do you have a medical condition?". I hesitated - I still remember it; I hesitated because I wondered whether this would be attributed to a medical condition.
I still ticked the box that I didn't and was gainfully employed for a number of years...'
Research participant

Despite progress over recent decades, workplaces are still predominantly designed for people without disabilities [279, 288]. From the outset (during the job-seeking process), my research found that people with dyslexia faced perceived discrimination, unfair judgments and lack of access to reasonable supports or adjustments during the screening and recruitment process. Until now, there has been minimal research that looks at the challenges faced by dyslexics when trying to find and gain employment. There has been a large body of research looking into recruitment barriers faced by those with other disabilities [288, 289], including autism [289-292]. Still, there has been limited research overseas, and none in Australia, that looks at job-seeking experiences of dyslexics until now. Finding job roles that align with our strengths and abilities can be difficult for dyslexics. In an ideal world, those with dyslexia would be able to take on positions that allow them to leverage their talents while minimising the impact of their dyslexia, but this is not so easy to do. As discussed earlier, many dyslexics are being under-employed compared to their education level.

Dyslexic individuals reported facing a range of barriers during the recruitment process, which can significantly impact their ability to secure employment. Traditional recruitment practices that require a high level of literacy skills, such as a cover letter, a resume, and selection criteria, can all present as barriers. Disorganised sentences and spelling and grammar mistakes can rule an individual out, as this can create a negative first impression with recruitment teams. Now, AI tools are being used to identify errors that can quickly rule dyslexic candidates out. My mum and friends would spend hours helping me craft my job applications, and it was so frustrating that I had to rely on their support all the time! Once an individual is ready to submit their application, they may then be faced with another barrier: Online Application Systems, which now require an individual to have a high level of digital literacy skills. Some dyslexics may face difficulties navigating complex online application systems, which often involve high levels of reading, following multiple steps, requiring precise data entry and then the system can time out! This can put those with dyslexia under significant time pressure, which can then affect processing speed, making it challenging for individuals to complete application processes. Leaving those with dyslexia feeling quite stressed about the job application process with a heightened sense of anxiety due to concerns about their written communication abilities.

These traditional processes potentially excludes not just those with dyslexia but also other candidates, such as those for whom English is a second language or who may have low digital literacy skills. I am all for streamlining processes and the use of recruitment systems, but you could be losing a potentially highly skilled pool of candidates without even knowing it. Yet there is so much that can be done to reduce this stress and enable those with dyslexia but for all candidates to perform at their best. It comes down to having more inclusive recruitment practices, and this is how we can do it. Let's look at some steps that can be taken to create more inclusive recruitment practices that will not just support dyslexic job seekers but can benefit all. This is not rocket science, and you may already be doing so of this work. The below may be adding to your toolbox, or you may not be, and this is the opportunity to start working towards more inclusive ways of recruiting that support all job seekers, not just those who are dyslexic.

6.2.1. Accessible role advertising:

- Add videos and audio records when advertising the role and the type of organisation it is, including values, business goals and other relevant information, to explain to a job seeker why they would want to work for your company.
- Use neuro-affirming language that avoids stigmatising or pathologising, such as replacing disorder with condition or difficulties with differences.
- Use correct terms such as autism instead of autism spectrum disorder.
- Some people like to use *Identity-first language*, such as I am dyslexic, while others might like to use person-first language. Person-first language emphasises the individual first and their neurodivergence second (e.g., 'person with dyslexia'). As you can see throughout this book, I have used both. If unsure just ask!

Include statements that showcase that your company is inclusive of neurodivergent employees, rather than a one-sentence statement stating you encourage those with disabilities to apply for job roles. Example of inclusive job advertisement Box 1.

6.2.2. Accessible Job Descriptions:

- Use plain language and avoid jargon in job descriptions.
- Provide information in a clear and organised format; dot points are always helpful
- Have text-to-speech functionality so individuals can listen to the job description, not just have to read it.

Have a video explaining the job description and providing information on the organisation's values and goals, for example.

6.2.3. Flexible Application Process:

- Allow for alternative application methods, such as video submissions, presentations or skills assessments, to showcase a candidate's abilities beyond traditional written materials.
- Provide extra time for completing assessments or applications if needed.

Are the other ways to capture experience apart from having a candidate submit a section criteria?

6.2.4. Clear Communication:

- Clearly communicate the recruitment process, including the steps involved and candidates' expectations.
- Have plain language statements that make it easy to understand what is expected of the job role.

Provide contact information for questions and support and encourage open communication.

At [Your Company Name], we are committed to fostering a workplace that values diversity and inclusivity. We recognise the unique strengths that individuals with dyslexia and other neurodivergences bring to the table, and we actively encourage applicants with dyslexia to apply for this position. We understand that traditional qualifications may not fully capture the talents of every candidate. If you have strong problem-solving skills, creative thinking and adaptability, we welcome your application.

At [Your Company Name], we provide different accommodations to suit your needs during the application and interview process. We believe that diversity enhances our team's innovation and success, and we look forward to welcoming individuals with dyslexia to contribute their valuable perspectives to our workplace.

6.2.5. Psychometric assessments

'. . . I failed the government test. After the test, two ladies sat in front of me and said, "You don't look dumb. We've never seen anybody fail a test as bad as this." And I said, "Well, I'm dyslexic," as my eyes dropped. It's hard [trying to] find another job. I applied for so many positions knowing that I have done this for over 30 years. And I can't get past the exam...'
Research participant

One of the most noticeable barriers identified in my research was the heavy reliance on psychometric testing during the recruitment process. These tests are not dyslexia-friendly, featuring questions that may need to be read with a written response with time limits that time you out. These tests create a considerable barrier for applicants with dyslexia. Time pressure can be particularly stressful for dyslexic individuals. They may require more time to process written information, and time constraints during assessments can put them at a disadvantage, leading to performance anxiety. My research found that even when dyslexics disclose their disability and ask for accommodations, they were not provided. 'Some were told, *just do your best.*' One research participant had a horrendous experience during a job interview:

We suggest that if your pre-hire practices do include assessments that reasonable accommodations are made for dyslexics, it's not cheating. If you had a blind candidate and you put them in front of a test, would you expect them to read the questions, or would you have accommodation in place to support them, so they are not disadvantaged? It's the same for dyslexics. If they must sit tests, can they have extra time? Is there an option for text-to-speech so the candidate can listen to the question? Sheppard-Jones et al (2021) suggests in their work that assessments be designed by employing a mixed methods approach. This involves utilising interviews and focus groups to ensure assessments that can be more inclusive, not only for neuro-atypical job seekers but for all individuals seeking employment.

6.2.6. Interview procedures

'...I disclosed in the interview that I had dyslexia and needed a computer to help me write down the answers. The recruiter looked at me and said, just try your best...'
Research participant

If the candidate is anything like me and struggles to navigate their way around, just getting to the interview can be mentally and emotionally taxing if we don't know the area well. I am constantly getting lost and must allow myself an extra thirty minutes to get lost, call for help, find where I need to go and then calm myself down. This can all add to the stress of the interview process.

Once in the interview, dyslexia can affect an individual's ability to organise thoughts and articulate ideas coherently, especially under pressure. This makes it more challenging to excel in interview situations, where effective communication is essential. The difficulties of organisation our thoughts can significantly heighten stress and anxiety, common emotional hurdles that many dyslexic job seekers face. You might be thinking, *well, everyone feels stressed and anxious in a job interview,* and this is true. However, when thinking of a dyslexic candidate they may have difficulty expressing themselves under pressure and feel anxious if they are to produce written information during the interview or sit a test, then the uncertainty and fear of whether to disclose their dyslexia can all create an additional layer of stress and pressure that those without a disability do not have to face. This additional stress can further hinder their performance during interviews and assessments.

Many individuals with dyslexia choose not to disclose their condition during the recruitment process due to concerns about stigma, bias and lack of understanding. This can make it challenging for recruiters to provide necessary accommodations and create an inclusive environment. In my research, I found that when dyslexics disclosed that they had a disability, they were not provided with appropriate reasonable adjustments. In my personal experience in job interview, I once disclosed I needed some additional editing support, and then I wasn't offered the salary they had advertised until they had determined *how much support I needed.* After my probation period, I told my then-manager I was dyslexic, and she said, *'I knew something was wrong with you!* It's important for recruitment teams to be trained on dyslexia and neurodivergence so they can provide appropriate accommodations and create a sense of psychological safety during the interview process to ensure a fair and inclusive experience.

To address these difficulties and create a more inclusive interview process, consider implementing the following adjustments:

Provide Questions in Advance: Offering questions beforehand allows dyslexic candidates to prepare and reduces the pressure associated with on-the-spot thinking.

Use Multiple Assessment Methods: Incorporate a variety of assessment methods, such as practical tasks, skills demonstrations and situational judgment tests, to evaluate candidates beyond traditional written or verbal responses.

Allow Extra Time: Provide additional time for written assessments or tasks, as dyslexic individuals may take longer to complete them.

Offer Alternative Communication Methods: Allow candidates to express themselves through alternative methods, such as diagrams, charts or presentations, instead of relying solely on verbal or written responses.

Create a Supportive Environment: Foster a supportive and understanding atmosphere during interviews, making it clear that accommodations are available and that the focus is on assessing skills and abilities.

By making these adjustments, employers can create a more inclusive interview experience for dyslexic individuals and ensure their true capabilities are assessed fairly. Employers also play a vital role by fostering inclusive recruitment practices and providing accommodations to ensure a level playing field for all candidates, including those with dyslexia. In Chapter 8, Universal Design Principles, you will find further information.

6.3. RETENTION

*'...I remember because I felt like walking out of a meeting – one guy said,
"If you're dyslexic, this won't make any sense to you" make it a joke of it
like you're stupid or something...'*
Research participant

Once recruited into a position, dyslexics may encounter significant and persistent challenges in fulfilling their work requirements due to systemic barriers within the organisation. You can't spend all your time and energy creating inclusive recruitment practices and then not have inclusive retention practices as well. You are setting the individual up to fail and you will see costly turnover rates when the individual quits or is terminated. Employee turnover is reported to have cost Australian businesses $3.8 billion over 12 months [293] - that's crazy!

The first 45 days of employment are a 'high-risk' period, with up to 20 per cent of new employees leaving during what's often referred to as the 'honeymoon' phase. According to research by Price Waterhouse Coopers (PWC), 23% of new employees in Australia leave their jobs within their first 12 months [293]. This highlights that the risk of turnover extends well beyond the initial onboarding period for all employees. Reasons employees may leave the job include being oversold and finding the reality of the role doesn't match the expectations set during recruitment, poor onboarding experience, lack of job role clarity,

poor management; whether it's micromanaging, unprepared managers or general management mishaps. No growth opportunities, where employees may realise there's no clear path for career advancement. Infrequent check-ins with a lack of regular feedback and communication can leave employees feeling unsupported and disconnected. Rigid workplace policies that don't support work-life balance or contribute to a hostile work environment can push employees out the door. Finally, insufficient support is when employees don't receive the support they need; they're more likely to look elsewhere [293].

Let's overlay this with the additional challenges those with dyslexia may face. As you would know by now, there is not enough research that exists in Australia, evaluating low literacy and numeracy skills caused by dyslexia within the workplace, until now. What international research tells us, is that effective communication across a variety of written mediums is an essential criterion in many workplace environments, and that when people with dyslexia enter the workforce, they must adapt to a complex environment with numerous demands, often with little to no support [211]. Those with dyslexia may struggle to meet workplace demands, where effective verbal and written communication skills are increasingly required. Specific problems those with dyslexia may face in the workplace, include overly complex tasks that increase workload stress, reliance on support from colleagues or family members at home, and challenges the physical working environment may present, such as background noise and other distractions [211, 281]. This can be further exacerbated by a mismatch between employees' abilities and employers' expectations [294], leading to a heightened risk of undue stress and anxiety, an employee not meeting work-based performance expectations, limited career prospects and compromised social and emotional well-being [158, 211, 273, 274, 295]

Challenges typically arise for dyslexics from structural obstacles within the organisation, such as a lack of established guidelines, practices, policies and procedures that are not inclusive of dyslexic employees and those with other neurodivergences, such as ADHD. An unsupportive or non-inclusive workplace culture can contribute to feelings of isolation and hinder professional growth. As a result, managers, human resources personnel and co-workers tend to have limited knowledge and awareness about dyslexia as a disability, despite it being the most prevalent disability in the workplace. This has a negative flow-on effect across the organisation and employee lifecycle.

Collegial relationships and supportive working environments are integral to managing job demands and encouraging people with dyslexia to undertake self-advocacy and help-seeking behaviours [296]. Yet the experience of my research indicated there is a considerable lack of awareness and understanding of dyslexia and its impact on workplace performance. Evidence from my research, and international studies, suggests that professional development and awareness-raising strategies are needed to address current knowledge deficits, and that meaningful effort is necessary for organisations to meet policy and legislative objectives of workplace inclusion [185, 297, 298]. Additionally, there are attitudinal challenges due to a lack of understanding and awareness, among employers and work colleagues, as to how the characteristics of dyslexia can affect workplace performance. For those with dyslexia, this can lead to feelings of discrimination and being stigmatised [274]. The cost of excessive work stress, such as feeling overwhelmed and emotionally exhausted, may have significant consequences for individuals and their organisations [299].

From the available literature, access to reasonable adjustments in the workplace is limited, posing another risk factor to employees and employers [27, 185, 287]. Likewise, receiving approval for reasonable adjustments is often not timely or forthcoming and is at managers' discretion rather than outlined in a policy. As you will see in Chapter 8, the process of accessing workplace accommodations can end up becoming a nightmare for the dyslexic employee who must disclose and get support from a variety of team members across operations, including IT, Finance, HR and often leadership. Insufficient access to assistive technology, such as speech-to-text software or dyslexia-friendly tools, may hinder productivity and efficiency especially if IT is blocking access due to the perception of potential security risks. This suggests that policies and procedures are insufficient to create inclusive practices for dyslexic employees, and there is no clear pathway for dyslexics to seek help from the operations team. This aligns with the work of Deacon et al. (2020), who found that having an unsupportive line manager could lead to job strain and individuals being fearful of seeking support. We will discuss this further in chapter 8. Furthermore, the stress associated with managing dyslexia in the workplace, coupled with a lack of awareness and understanding of the difficulties associated with dyslexia and the potential misconceptions about abilities, can contribute to burnout and decreased job satisfaction. This is discussed in detail in Chapter 7 - Workplace well-being.

By addressing these retention barriers and fostering an inclusive workplace culture, employers can create an environment where dyslexic individuals feel valued, supported and able to thrive in their careers.

6.4. CAREER PROGRESSION

'...I get depressed about it sometimes. It's probably cost me promotion-wise a few times as well, I think. Going through that again now. I think they think you're not capable of it. It's come back as "you're not confident" or "you're not capable". It sort of looks like that to the people above you – it's frustrating for me as I know I am capable, It's pretty depressing ...'
Research participant

There is limited research on the area of career progression for those with dyslexia. My research indicated that there were many obstacles for dyslexics who were trying to enter the labour market after completing a degree, to find employment or progress in their careers.

Career progression for dyslexic employees can be influenced by a combination of factors stemming from traditional recruitment practices, including psychometric testing. When some of the individuals disclosed their dyslexia, they felt they were then perceived differently, and it appeared that their managers saw them to be less competent and, therefore, unable to progress in their careers. Others felt they had hit the 'glass ceiling' and could not proceed any further within the company they were currently working for. Perhaps if these employees had the right workplace accommodations in place, they would have been about to demonstrate their strengths and their full potential. Instead, they have been left to feel disappointed, frustrated and depressed that they are stuck in certain role, underemployed based on their qualifications or struggling to find employment.

We are seeing a lot of research undertaken within the autistic community about unemployment and underemployment, and I strongly believe much more research needs to be done for the dyslexic community. I work with many dyslexics who are unable to progress in their careers, are performance-managed out because of their dyslectic and are unemployed and unable to access appropriate neuro-affirming services to help them gain meaningful employment. There is enormous untapped potential sitting in and out of organisations, and this, frankly, isn't good enough. The ongoing financial barriers and mental health challenges linked to unemployment, underemployment and poor working conditions for those with dyslexia cannot and should not be ignored any longer.

6.5. CONCLUSION

Congratulations on getting through this mammoth chapter. After reviewing this chapter, I hope you can see that it is imperative for employers and companies to align inclusive workplace practices with their commitments, particularly regarding individuals with dyslexia and other neurodivergences. The financial impact of employee turnover, ranging from 30% to 150% of their salary, underscores the substantial burden on businesses. The challenges faced by individuals with dyslexia throughout the employment lifecycle, highlight the urgent need for a more empathetic approach and improved workplace policies.

The lack of extensive research on dyslexia-specific challenges in graduating and gaining employment in Australia emphasises the need for increased awareness and targeted education and training across education, higher education and employment. These stories aren't being heard. There is silence, and this must change. A multi-layered approach is needed within organisations, starting by removing traditional recruitment practices that create unnecessary barriers and enabling access to reasonable adjustments during the hiring, which will, in turn, create a more equitable recruitment process.

Internal workplace policies often fall short in addressing the needs of individuals with dyslexia, leading to stress and hindered performance. My research emphasises the importance of understanding, 'reasonable adjustments,' and supportive working environments. Retention barriers for individuals with dyslexia require a multifaceted approach, including education, flexible work arrangements, accommodations, mentorship programs, and inclusive workplace policies. By embracing these measures, employers can create an environment where dyslexic individuals feel valued, supported and empowered, aligning with policy objectives and contributing to overall well-being and success.

KEY TAKE-HOME MESSAGES
Urgent Need for Inclusivity: Dyslexic individuals' experiences in the recruitment and onboarding processes underscore the immediate need

for more inclusive workplace practices. Discrimination, lack of support, and limited research in this area emphasise the urgency of addressing dyslexia-specific challenges.

Unique Challenges Require Specific Attention: While there is extensive research on recruitment barriers for individuals with disabilities, the unique challenges faced by dyslexic individuals necessitate targeted attention. Employers should recognise and address these challenges to create a more equitable job-seeking environment.

Revamping Job Advertising Practices: To attract and support dyslexic individuals, employers should incorporate neuro-affirming language, provide clear information about the organisation's values, and actively showcase inclusivity in their job advertisements. A more transparent and accessible approach can contribute to a more diverse applicant pool.

Universal Design Principles across recruitment processes: Employers should look at ways to try and incorporate the seven principles of universal design, ensuring flexibility, minimal errors and inclusive development in psychometric assessments and recruitment processes. A mixed methods approach, including interviews and focus groups, can help design assessments that cater to the diverse traits of neurodivergent job seekers.

Inclusive Interview Practices: Recognising the impact of dyslexia on communication and organisation, employers should make adjustments to the interview process. Providing questions in advance, using multiple assessment methods, offering extra time and allowing alternative communication methods, create a supportive environment for dyslexic individuals to showcase their abilities.

Encouraging Disclosure and Providing Support: Employers play a pivotal role in fostering an inclusive environment by encouraging candidates to disclose their dyslexia without fear of discrimination.

Providing necessary accommodations, educating hiring teams and consistently offering support throughout the recruitment journey are crucial steps toward a more inclusive workplace.

Persisting Workplace Challenges: Individuals with dyslexia encounter significant and persistent challenges in the workplace, often stemming from a lack of awareness, understanding and supportive policies.

Structural Obstacles and Limited Awareness: The absence of established guidelines and practices, coupled with limited awareness among managers and co-workers, contributes to difficulties for dyslexic employees.

Inadequate Workplace Policies: Internal workplace policies often lack sensitivity to the distinctive experiences of employees with dyslexia, leading to the need for self-devised strategies. Policies do not effectively support inclusive working environments.

Need for 'Reasonable Adjustments': Providing workplace adjustments is not about doing a *nice thing*, it's a legal requirement to support employees with dyslexia. Workplaces must develop a clear understanding of what constitutes a 'reasonable adjustment' and provide appropriate support, including access to assistive technologies, coaching and peer support.

Lack of Collegial Understanding: Despite the importance of collegial relationships, the research reveals a significant lack of awareness and understanding of dyslexia's impact on workplace performance among colleagues.

Retention Barriers and Strategies: Specific challenges, including communication difficulties, reading and comprehension issues, and limited access to assistive technology, contribute to retention barriers. Strategies such as education, flexible work arrangements, accommodations, mentorship programs and inclusive workplace policies can address these barriers.

Promoting Inclusive Workplace Cultures: Employers should focus on fostering an inclusive workplace culture by educating the workforce, adapting performance appraisal methods and promoting policies that recognise and support neurodiversity.

Diversity as a Strength: Embracing diversity, including neurodiversity, contributes to a richer and more innovative workplace. Employers who actively address the challenges faced by dyslexic individuals, not only enhance the recruitment experience for these individuals but also tap into a unique pool of talent that can bring valuable perspectives to the organisation.

Well-Being and Professional Growth: Addressing dyslexia-related challenges is crucial for enhancing well-being, preventing burnout and unlocking the full potential of dyslexic individuals for professional growth.

Continuous Professional Development and Awareness: Professional development and awareness-raising strategies are necessary to bridge knowledge gaps and meet policy and legislative objectives of workplace inclusion.

In summary, creating a truly inclusive workplace for individuals with dyslexia requires a concerted effort to address awareness gaps, implement supportive policies and provide the necessary accommodations. By doing so, employers can not only enhance the work experience for dyslexic individuals but also contribute to a more diverse, resilient and successful organisational culture.

CASE STUDY 1 – RECRUITMENT

Jo, having experienced three months of unemployment, finally lands an interview opportunity for the position of a customer service officer at a local government council. This prospect excites Jo, as the role promises the potential for stable, ongoing employment - a welcome change from the short-term contracts that have characterised their recent work history. However, the constant cycle of job applications, involving detailed written submissions, such as selection criteria and cover letters, has been a source of frustration and anxiety for Jo.

Navigating the intricacies of these short-term contracts is particularly challenging for Jo due to their dyslexia, adding an extra layer of stress. The need for meticulous proofreading before submitting applications and the recurring financial insecurity associated with short-term roles, intensify the pressure Jo feels to excel in the upcoming interview.

Anticipating potential challenges in the new role, Jo acknowledges the necessity of support during the initial months due to their dyslexia. With this in mind, Jo decides to disclose their condition to the HR consultant during the interview, a crucial step towards securing the understanding and assistance they may require.

On the day of the interview, Jo takes proactive measures, leaving home an hour early to account for their tendency to get lost in unfamiliar places. The additional time allows Jo to navigate the location, calm the ensuing stress, and compose themselves before the interview. Jo's partner, a steadfast source of support, aids in interview preparation, extending their assistance beyond the professional realm to encompass daily tasks like finding car keys and managing finances - areas where Jo grapples, particularly in issues related to numbers.

As Jo steps into the interview room, they are met with three individuals seated at the table - the HR consultant, the line manager, and a manager from another team. Anxiety creeps in, evident in the beads of sweat forming on Jo's forehead and the trembling of their hands. Throughout the interview, Jo shares their experiences and articulates what they are eager to contribute to the role. However, the pivotal moment arrives when Jo decides to disclose their dyslexia, momentarily casting a hush over the room. This disclosure, intended to foster understanding, takes an unexpected turn.

Following the interview, the HR consultant requests Jo to step into the next room for psychometric testing. Dread sets in as Jo realises the challenges that lie ahead; past experiences have shown that these tests, coupled with the limitations imposed by dyslexia, have resulted in missed job opportunities. As Jo sits down for the testing, they muster the courage to request additional time and the use of text-to-speech features. Unfortunately, their plea is met with a disheartening response from the HR consultant, who denies these accommodations, citing concerns about creating an 'unfair advantage' and urging Jo to simply 'try their best.'

This denial sets the stage for heightened stress and uncertainty, underscoring the ongoing challenges individuals with dyslexia face in navigating professional opportunities and the need for greater awareness and accommodation in the hiring process.

Dyslexic employees may find different types of working environments stressful. One such environment is the open office where they may be sensitive to background noise and get sensory overload. They may struggle with concentration and become easily distracted in an open-planned office where people are talking around them, or there might be people sitting on Teams or Zoom meetings and others taking phone calls. If someone is speaking to them and there is background noise, they may find it hard to focus on what is being said. The other person may become frustrated if it appears they are not paying attention, especially if they need to be following instructions and/or participating in the conversation. Since COVID, those with dyslexia might find the transition back to the office especially difficult, as they could control their working environment at home, and now, they are unable to do this in an office setting.

Another example is the use of technology. In order to survive and flourish, many dyslexics have become tech savvy. But for some, technology can be a cause of frustration and stress. If a dyslexic uses different devices at home and at work, such as a Mac and a PC, having to alternate between the two could prove difficult. They may feel frustrated having to learn different ways of working to make the different technologies compatible with each other. All of this can play havoc for a dyslexic, who might be trying to read and/or write and can lead to the building of anxiety and stress.

CASE STUDIES

At the end of this chapter there are three case studies (pseudonyms used) which highlight how changes in the environment, job role or manager can have a significant impact, taking a mental toll on dyslexic employees and those who work with them. These case studies are drawn from my research.

Case study 1: Navigating the working environment: The struggles of Morris Burn

This case study highlights the experiences of Morris Burn, an employee with dyslexia working at a call-centre officer in a large Telco. Morris had been working in a new role at the call centre for six months and although he enjoyed the role, he had not disclosed his dyslexia to anyone in his workplace. The environment was very noisy, as people were on phones all day. It was difficult to concentrate with all the background noise. Morris started to realise, that for the first time in a job role he was struggling, and that his dyslexia was affecting him severely. He couldn't meet his KPIs, like everyone else, and was slower, needing more time. Morris realised he was feeling significant sensory overload. He felt an inability to concentrate, to be able to read information off a page or be able to hear information clearly, and then be able to transcribe it; there was a lot of fuzz in his head. He couldn't read things as clearly and pick up every word, needing to re-read documents repeatedly to get the correct information. It meant he was taking a lot longer to do the things that should only take, perhaps, a couple of minutes to do. He had never felt sensory overload before in previous roles. Overall, he felt he was struggling in general. It was making him feel quite unhappy, uneasy and he was fearing going to work. He started to question his career path. He was fearful that he may lose his job if he didn't disclose his dyslexia to his manager.

RESOLUTION

In response to Morris' challenges, a proactive approach was taken to address the issues he faced in the call centre environment. A confidential conversation was initiated with Morris to understand the specific difficulties he encountered. It was during this discussion that Morris disclosed his dyslexia, explaining how the noise in the call centre exacerbated his sensory overload, impacting his ability to meet performance targets.

To facilitate a more supportive work environment, reasonable accommodations were implemented. Morris was provided noise-cancelling headphones to mitigate the impact of ambient noise, creating a quieter space for him to focus on his tasks. Additionally, he was granted additional time allowances to meet his KPIs, recognising the extra effort required due to his dyslexia.

Further, a training program on dyslexia awareness and support was introduced for all employees within the call centre. This aimed to not only to raise awareness about dyslexia but also to foster a more inclusive workplace culture, and encourage other employees with dyslexia and other neurodivergences to come forward for support.

6.6. CONCLUSION:

Through these interventions, Morris experienced a positive shift in his work environment. The noise-cancelling headphones significantly reduced sensory overload, allowing him to concentrate better and enhance his task performance. The additional time allowances provided the necessary flexibility for Morris to meet his KPIs, without compromising the quality of his work. The dyslexia awareness training contributed to a more understanding and empathetic workplace, diminishing the stigma associated with disclosing neurodiverse conditions. Morris' disclosure of dyslexia to his manager resulted in a supportive and collaborative atmosphere, where his unique needs were acknowledged and accommodated. Morris took the lead on creating a Neurodivergent Network within the company that offered peer support and access to services within the company, championed by Morris' manager at a leadership level.

Ultimately, Morris' job satisfaction improved, and his fear of losing his job diminished, as the workplace embraced inclusivity. This case serves as a testament to the positive outcomes achievable through proactive measures and a commitment to creating an accommodating and supportive work environment for individuals with dyslexia.

ACCESSIBILITY ONBOARDING CHECK LIST			
Do you need any of the following resources or tools to support you in your day-to-day work?			
Tool	Yes	No	Unsure
Microsoft Immersion set up			
Grammarly			
Text to speech			
Mind mapping app			
Access to a white board			

Fathom or other note taking software			
Remarkable note pad			
Goblin Tool, Chat GPT, Wordtune			
Work environments	Yes	No	Unsure
Noise cancelling headphones			
Working from home			
Ability to change the lights			
Structuring of your working day	Yes	No	Unsure
Start work early and finish early			
Start work late and finish late			
Extra breaks in my day			
Extra time in the day allocated for tasks such as reading and writing			
How I like to work	Yes	No	Unsure
I don't like being interrupted.			
I like to plan my day; I don't like surprises.			
I like to be fully prepared and trained before undertaking a new task			
I need to structure to ensure I can meet deadlines			
I like instructions:			
verbal format			
written format			

watch a video			
I like to have a peer proofread important documents for me			
I like to have colleague support when learning new tasks			
I like to work in a team			
I like to work independently			
Workplace strengths	Yes	No	Unsure
Creative thinker			
Problem solver			
Big picture thinker			
Strategic			
Fine detailed			
Love numbers and spreadsheets			
Story telling			
Critical thinking			
Public speaking			
Networking and collaborating			

Chapter 7
WORKPLACE WELL-BEING AND BURNOUT

"When you are constantly stressed about how to fit in and do your job as a neurodivergent person in a neurotypical world, the stress can have serious consequences."

- Dr. Pope-Ruark, Psychology Today

In this chapter, we will unpack the issues of psychosocial hazards and burnout in the workplace. The aim of this chapter is for us to become proactive in mitigating psychosocial hazards for neurodivergent employees. In Australia, work-related psychological conditions have been increasing, leading to extended absences from work [293] and, as such, are cause for concern for both employees and employers. When psychosocial hazards are not addressed, it can lead to burnout. Burnout is a growing concern, as highlighted by a 2022 Microsoft Work Trend Index study, which found that Australian workers have the highest burnout rates globally. In Australia, 61% of workers reported experiencing burnout, compared to the global average of 48% [294]. Similarly, a recent global study by UiPath revealed that 82% of Australian knowledge workers (e.g., ICT Professionals,) feel burnt out, with 36% feeling very or extremely burnt out, surpassing all other surveyed countries [295]. The economic impact is significant, with burnout and stress-related absenteeism costing the Australian economy an estimated $14 billion annually [294].

Although everyone is at risk of psychosocial hazards and burnout in the workplace, those with dyslexia and other neurodivergences are at greater risk due to the complex nature of their difficulties, especially when not supported. Let's dive into this further now, looking at psychosocial hazards in the workplace and the Safe Work Australia, Managing Psychosocial Hazards at Work: Code of Practice. We will look at what burnout is and how it can present, using the Job Demands-Resources Model of Burnout to illustrate this in day-to-day practice for dyslexic employees and their workplaces.

7.1. PSYCHOLOGICAL SAFETY IN THE WORKPLACE

Psychological safety refers to a work environment where all employees feel comfortable and confident to express their opinions, ideas, and concerns and even make mistakes without fear of negative consequences [296]. In psychologically safe workplaces, people are encouraged to collaborate, learn from their experiences and contribute to the organisation's growth and innovation. Implementing effective strategies in the workplace can lead to a reduction in absenteeism, workplace incidents, workers' compensation claims, staff turnover and the costs associated with recruitment and training [297].

Psychosocial hazards on the other hand, have the potential to inflict both psychological and physical harm. On average, psychological injuries arising from work have lengthier recovery periods, elevated costs and necessitate more extensive time off from work [298]. Effectively managing the risks linked to psychosocial hazards not only safeguards employees, but also reduces the disturbances tied to employee turnover and absenteeism [298]. Furthermore, it holds the potential to enhance overall organisational performance and productivity. Psychosocial hazards can come from:

the design or management of work

- a work environment
- plant (e.g. equipment) at a workplace, or
- workplace interactions or behaviours [297, 298].

Some of the key psychosocial hazards we identified in our research for dyslexic employees that fall under the *Managing Psychosocial Hazards at work: Code of Practice 2022*, include:

- High job demands where an employee is facing intense or sustained high mental, physical or emotional effort required to do the job.
- Low job resources or control, such as employees having little control over aspects of the work, including how or when the job is done.
- Poor support
- Poor organisational change management, bullying, harassment and conflict, or poor workplace relationships and interactions.

Organisations now must, so far as is reasonably practicable, ensure workers and other people are not exposed to risks to their psychological or physical health and safety. Employers have a duty of care and must work towards eliminating psychosocial risks in the workplace [298]. In the fast-paced, changing work environment, the ongoing work demands, tasks, and responsibilities combined with unsupported dyslexic difficulties can start to create mental fatigue and cognitive overload, which is the precursor to job burnout. Let's explore burnout now.

7.2. BURNOUT

You can't pour from an empty glass.
Dr Malvika Behal

Psychosocial hazards in the workplace can lead to workplace stress and, eventually, burnout. According to the World Health Organisation (WHO), burnout is a syndrome that arises from chronic job-related stressors that have not been effectively managed. Burnout is classified as a medical condition that is characterised by three elements: feelings of energy depletion or exhaustion; a growing mental distance from one's job, accompanied by feelings of negativism or cynicism towards one's work; and, a reduction in professional efficacy [299]. 'Burnout refers specifically to phenomena in the occupational context and should not be applied to describe experiences in other areas of life [299].'

Burnout can also significantly impact an individual's personal life, manifesting through various psychological and behavioural traits, such as:

- Low levels of self-esteem: Individuals may struggle with feelings of inadequacy and self-doubt.
- External focus of control: There is a tendency to believe that outside forces, rather than personal actions, dictate outcomes.
- Low levels of sense of coherence: A diminished ability to perceive life as comprehensible, manageable and meaningful.
- Alexithymia: Difficulty in identifying and expressing emotions.
- High levels of neuroticism: A predisposition to experience negative

emotions like anxiety, anger and depression [294].

These characteristics not only exacerbate the experience of burnout but also affect overall well-being and quality of life. When I did a literature search on dyslexia and burnout, I found one explicit research paper - it was mine! Although excited to see it (and we will investigate further), it was also very concerning. There were a few articles on burnout and dyslexic students, but *what about the working adults?* I cry! And then I found more of my research ... but I digress. When I looked up autism and burnout, I found twenty articles, and it kept going. I then looked at ADHD and burnout; not as many as autism but still a lot more than on dyslexia. If you do a web search, it's even bigger, overwhelming compared to what you find on dyslexia, indicating we need so much more research into this and the interconnectedness of co-occurring conditions. Let's look at what my research found using the Job-Demands Resource Model of Burnout.

7.3. DYSLEXIA AND THE JOB DEMANDS RESOURCE MODEL OF BURNOUT (JD-R MODEL)

Graph .1. Dyslexia and the spike profile

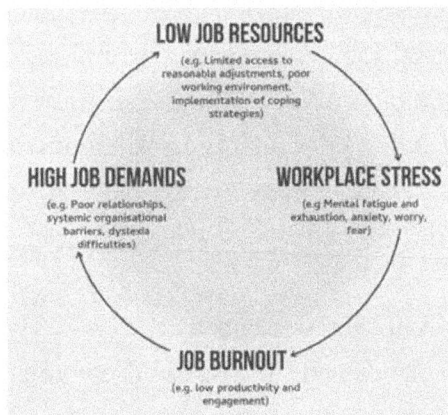

LOW JOB RESOURCES
(e.g. Limited access to reasonable adjustments, poor working environment, implementation of coping strategies)

HIGH JOB DEMANDS
(e.g. Poor relationships, systemic organisational barriers, dyslexia difficulties)

WORKPLACE STRESS
(e.g Mental fatigue and exhaustion, anxiety, worry, fear)

JOB BURNOUT
(e.g. low productivity and engagement)

Australian workers reported the highest burnout rates in the world. An alarming 61% of Australian workers reported experiencing burnout, compared to the global average of 48% [294]. The JD-R Model looks at the link between job characteristics (demands and resources) and employee well-being (burnout and engagement) (Figure 12.) [300]. It is a validated model, which uses both surveys and individual feedback from employees, and has been used in a variety of studies to evaluate and predict important organisational outcomes across several industries [300-304]. The JD-R model highlights that all occupations bring with them specific risk factors that are linked with job stress, leading to job burnout. Job burnout is described as 'a chronic state of work-related psychological stress that is characterised by exhaustion (i.e., feeling emotionally drained and used up), mental distancing (i.e., cynicism and lack of enthusiasm), and reduced personal efficacy (i.e., doubting one's competence and contribution at work)'[305]. The JD-R model distinguishes two kinds of characteristics related to burnout and work engagement; job demands and job resources [306].

Job demands are the 'physical, psychological, social or organisational aspects of the job that require sustained physical and/or psychological (cognitive and emotional) effort or skills, and are therefore associated with certain physiological and/or psychological costs' [306]. The negative costs of job demands may be a result of instances, such as an unfavourable physical environment, intense work pressure and emotionally demanding jobs, such as interactions with patients.

Job resources are the 'physical, psychological, social or organisational aspects of the job that are either/or:

- functional in achieving work goals
- reduce job demands and the associated physiological and psychological costs

- stimulate personal growth, learning and development [306].

Furthermore, the JD–R model also includes two sets of risk factors: health impairment process and motivational process. Each may contribute to 'job strain and motivation.' In relation to health impairment processes, 'poorly designed jobs and high job demands (e.g., work overload or emotional demands) may exhaust an employee's mental and physical resources, leading to the depletion of energy (i.e., a state of exhaustion) and, hence, to health problems with job demands leading to burnout [307].

The motivational process is assumed to link job resources with organisational outcomes (e.g., turnover intention) through strengthening the commitment of employees to achieve the task/organisational goals. Motivation improves when job resources are used for positive feedback or ensuring employees are engaged in wanting to complete the task well [306].

Additionally, we felt it was important to include Personal Resources that form part of chapter 8 as an expansion of the JD-R Model, based on the work of Xanthopoulou, Bakker, Demerouti and Schaufeli (2009). Xanthopoulou et al (2009; p. 236) define personal resources as *positive self-evaluations that are linked to resiliency and refer to individuals' sense of their ability to control and impact upon their environment successfully.'* Examples of personal resources can include self-efficacy, optimism and organisation-based self-esteem [305].

As the central function of many workplaces is productivity outcomes, organisations tend to be driven by factors such as market force needs, and this is possibly less suited to accommodate dyslexic individuals [308]. In contrast, there has been a slow but increasing focus on the psychological risks and educational needs of dyslexic individuals who are still at school or in post-secondary education [94, 101, 206]. Additionally, legislative policy in Australia and overseas has been developed to ensure those with dyslexia are covered under several federal and state Acts. Yet, despite the ratification of such Acts and disability policies aimed at reducing discrimination, a commitment to the inclusion of individuals with diverse needs, such as dyslexia, is not as well-established or understood in Australian workplaces [309].

Prior to entering the workforce, individuals with dyslexia inevitably have a history of difficulty with learning, which began in childhood. These difficulties may or may not have been formally diagnosed. Recollections from childhood may include struggles with reading, writing, spelling and maths, as well as adverse emotional experiences such as trauma, abuse and discrimination [310]. Many children and adolescents have expressed, and described, a variety of negative experiences and emotions during their education, including disappointment, shame, frustration, embarrassment, sadness, depression, anxiety, anger and low self-esteem [32, 94, 310]. Those with dyslexia can transfer the negative experiences they encountered as a child into adulthood, no matter how long ago they occurred [97, 139, 310].

7.4. DYSLEXIA AND WORK-RELATED PSYCHOLOGICAL DISTRESS AND BURNOUT

Figure 12. Workplace psychological safety

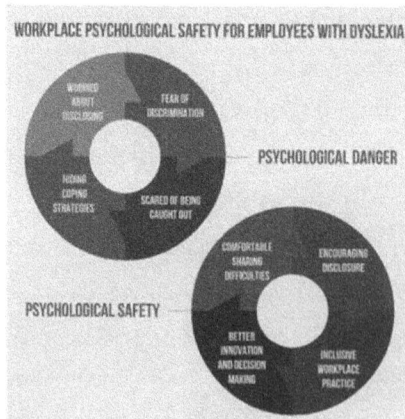

As mentioned, work-related psychosocial conditions are costing individuals and workplaces lots of money. The evidence to date suggests that individuals with dyslexia are vulnerable to personal and psychological stress at work [58, 144, 212, 311], and, unlike elsewhere, the workplace experiences of dyslexic adults have received very little attention in Australia.

The cost of excessive work stress, such as feeling cognitive overload and ongoing mental exhaustion, may have significant consequences for dyslexic individuals and their organisations [312]. Employee well-being plays a crucial role in how an organisation performs. When all employees, not just dyslexics experience autonomy at work, have supportive colleagues and managers, and have access to reasonable adjustments, they are intrinsically motivated to achieve their work goals [58, 212].

Research tells us the enduring and recurrent challenges encountered by individuals with dyslexia can provoke adverse emotional states, substantiated by the findings of prior local studies and international investigations [31, 212, 260, 313, 314]. These mental health issues can impact the ability to acquire a job, and once acquired, can affect the ability to stay in employment. To compensate for their difficulties, employees with dyslexia often apply considerable coping strategies [163, 277, 315], such as working longer hours, using templates or checklists, colour coding and using assistive technology [73, 186, 277, 312, 316]. Like my findings, the research tells us that people with dyslexia often feel they have no choice but to develop their own strategies and coping mechanisms when in a working environment that feels unsafe for disclosing their disability. This can lead to higher rates of workplace stress and lead to significant mental fatigue, feelings of isolation, lack of support and high anxiety [97, 230, 260, 277].

Failing to address the additional stressors that dyslexic employees are often placed under in the work context is a disservice, not only to the employees themselves but to employers and organisations. We know that people with dyslexia make a significant contribution to the community and have many strengths [194, 266]. Making reasonable adjustments in the workplace allows organisations to better harness those strengths and mitigate some of the mental health issues that people with dyslexia may experience.

Individuals with dyslexia may be more susceptible to burnout due to the additional challenges their dyslexia can cause when unsupported in a workplace setting. I have mentioned many of these factors above, such as increased cognitive load when having to rely heavily on their working memory, impacting executive functioning skills and leading to mental fatigue. Chronic stress and anxiety result from the constant struggle to meet academic or work expectations. Repeated experiences of failure or criticism can impact self-esteem and contribute to feelings of inadequacy, while insufficient accommodations and understanding from educators, employers and peers can exacerbate stress levels, all of which can lead to burnout.

7.5. MITIGATING PSYCHOSOCIAL HAZARDS AND BURNOUT FOR DYSLEXIC INDIVIDUALS

'...Being dyslexic my brain is scrambly and so managing priorities of conflicting pressures, you've got multiple tasks with the burden of oh my God I've got to write that and then I've got to edit it and how do I get it done in time with influx of work at the same time to just the mental load that that has on someone who struggles to organise thoughts, prioritise, juggle the plethora of electricity parts and it's an enormous mental load...'
Research participant

Okay, so we now have a good understanding that employers have a responsibility to create a psychologically safe work environment for all employees. Based on my research, here are some suggestions that you, as the employer, can do to reduce the risk of psychosocial hazards related to dyslexia. Some of these strategies you will already be doing because it's best practice for all staff, with just a few additional items for your dyslexic and/or other neurodivergent employees.

Raise Awareness: Provide training and information sessions for all employees to raise awareness about dyslexia and promote understanding. Improved working relationships support a strength-based approach and create empathic, psychologically safe environments.

Easy access to reasonable adjustments: Engage in open conversations with dyslexic employees to identify workplace adjustments that can ease the challenges their disability may give rise to, such as providing assistive technology, extending deadlines or offering alternative communication methods.

Flexible Communication Channels: Foster a culture that encourages diverse communication channels beyond written formats. Verbal discussions, one-on-one meetings and visual aids can accommodate different communication preferences.

Clear Expectations: Set realistic expectations and clear guidelines for tasks, ensuring that dyslexic individuals understand their responsibilities and feel confident in meeting them.

Mentorship and Support Networks: Establish mentorship programs that connect dyslexic employees with peers who have successfully navigated similar challenges. This can provide a sense of guidance and belonging. Peer support and mentoring programs are valuable additions to the workplace. Many organisations now have Ability committees or DEI working groups that can support dyslexic employees.

Performance Feedback: Offer constructive and supportive feedback that acknowledges their strengths and provides guidance on areas for improvement.

Addressing the unique challenges faced by individuals with dyslexia is crucial in reducing the risk of psychosocial hazards and burnout. Implementing supportive strategies and creating inclusive working environments will enhance productivity and improve the mental health and well-being of your workforce; it's a win-win for everyone,

Supporting yourself as a dyslexic

For you, the dyslexic, we touch on self-care in chapter 9 but here is a quick reminder of what can help you reduce burnout. These are no brainers we all know that we should be doing, so these are gentle reminders. Practicing regular physical exercise, mindfulness and relaxation techniques can help manage stress and burnout. Ensuring adequate sleep and maintaining a healthy diet supports overall well-being. Exploring accommodations such as extended deadlines or assistive technology, utilising tools like planners, calendars and task management apps can help organise tasks and deadlines, breaking tasks into smaller, manageable steps to avoid feeling overwhelmed. Consulting with mental health professionals for therapy and counselling, or your workplace EAP or our 1800 13 NEAP (6327) service, can help you with strategies that can ease work-related challenges and feelings of burnout.

7.6. CONCLUSION

The JD-R Model serves as a valuable framework for understanding the intricate relationship between job characteristics, employee well-being and organisational outcomes for those with dyslexia. It emphasises the impact of job demands and resources on burnout and work engagement, recognising the unique risk factors associated with different occupations. The model's incorporation of health impairment and motivational processes underscores the dual nature of its applicability, addressing both the negative consequence of job demands and the positive outcomes linked to job resources.

The identification of psychosocial hazards, particularly in the context of dyslexic individuals in the workplace, further highlights the importance of managing job demands and resources. High job demands, low job resources, poor support and challenges related to organisational change can contribute to psychological distress and job burnout. The legal landscape also plays a crucial role, with employers having a duty of care to eliminate or minimise psychosocial risks and ensure the psychological safety and well-being of employees under work health and safety laws. Additionally, the consideration of personal resources, such as self-efficacy, optimism and organisational-based self-esteem, expands the JD-R Model's scope and recognises the significance of the individual with dyslexia strengths in navigating workplace challenges.

In the broader context of work-related psychological conditions, dyslexic individuals in Australia face unique challenges that require understanding and attention. Employers need to understand that all employees can face psychosocial risks, but when unsupported, those with dyslexia often deal with bigger challenges because of their condition. Employers need to take proactive measures to address this. Emphasising the need for organisational awareness, responsive support systems and a commitment to psychological safety is good for all. By understanding and addressing psychosocial hazards, organisations can not only protect their employees from harm but also enhance overall performance and productivity and reduce risks associated with these hazards, contributing to a more diverse and resilient workforce.

KEY TAKE-HOME MESSAGES

Psychological Safety and Well-being: Psychological safety in the workplace promotes an environment where employees feel comfortable expressing themselves without fear of negative consequences. Effectively managing psychosocial hazards is essential for safeguarding employees, reducing turnover and enhancing overall organisational performance.

Psychosocial Hazards and Burnout are Critical Issues: Addressing psychosocial hazards in the workplace is essential to prevent burnout, especially for neurodivergent employees. In Australia, the rise in work-related psychological conditions, including burnout, is a significant concern, with economic implications totalling billions annually!

Increased Vulnerability for Neurodivergent Employees: Neurodivergent individuals, such as those with dyslexia, are at a higher risk of experiencing burnout due to the unique challenges they face. These challenges often stem from high job demands, low job resources and a lack of adequate support and accommodations due to low levels of psychological safety.

Psychological Safety is Key: Creating a psychologically safe work environment is crucial. This involves fostering a culture where employees feel comfortable expressing themselves and are supported in their roles, reducing the risk of burnout. The benefits are endless, including a decrease in absenteeism, workplace incidents, workers' compensation claims, staff turnover and costs associated with recruitment and training due to enhanced staff retention and fewer customer complaints [297].

JD-R Model Significance: The JD-R Model is a validated framework that links job characteristics (demands and resources) to employee well-being, specifically burnout and engagement. It distinguishes job demands, resources and personal resources, offering insights into the complex interplay between work-related factors and psychological outcomes. My research is the first of its kind to link the JD-R Model of burnout with dyslexic employees.

The JD-R Model as a Framework: The Job Demands-Resources (JD-R) Model is a valuable tool for understanding how job demands and resources impact burnout and employee well-being. For dyslexic employees, excessive job demands without sufficient resources can lead to burnout, making it essential for employers to provide the necessary support.

Importance of Personal Resources: Personal resources, such as self-efficacy and resilience, play a critical role in mitigating burnout. For neurodivergent employees, enhancing these resources through targeted support can significantly improve their ability to manage work-related stress.

Need for Targeted Research and Support: The lack of research on dyslexia and burnout in the workplace highlights the need for more attention to this issue. Employers must be proactive in addressing the specific needs of dyslexic employees to prevent burnout and foster a more inclusive work environment.

Mitigation Strategies: Employers can mitigate psychosocial hazards and burnout by raising awareness, offering reasonable adjustments, providing clear expectations and promoting an inclusive culture. These strategies not only benefit dyslexic employees but also enhance overall organisational performance.

RESOURCES

There are a huge number of resources you can find, so we are listing just a few to help you on your journey of discovery and understanding. You can find more information at re:think dyslexia.com.au. If you found any of this content distressing, please seek support:

- Lifeline on 13 11 14
- Beyond Blue - counsellor on 1300 22 4636
- NEAP Neurodivergent Employment Assistance Program on 1800 13 6327

People at Work, Australia government initiative

The "People at Work" survey is a free, validated tool designed to assess common psychosocial hazards in the Australian workplace. As part of a comprehensive five-step process, the survey helps you identify, assess and manage risks to psychological health at work [296]. The provided resources guide you through:

Preparing for and implementing the "People at Work" survey

Interpreting the survey results, and

Taking appropriate action based on those results.

Upon completing the survey, you'll receive a report that compares your organisation's results with industry benchmarks across Australia [296].

Further information can be found https://www.peopleatwork.gov.au/

RESEARCH

Wissell, S., Karimi, L. & Serry, T. Furlong, L & Hudson, H. (2022) 'You don't look dyslexic': Using the Job Demands - Resource model to explore workplace experiences of Australian adults with dyslexia. International Journal of Environmental Research and Public Health. S Ed. doi.org/10.3390/ijerph191710719

Books, podcasts and support

- Banishing Burnout: Six Strategies for Improving Your Relationship with Work by Michael P. Leiter and Christina Maslach
- The Resilient Practitioner: Burnout Prevention and Self-Care Strategies for Counselors, Therapists, Teachers and Health Professionals by Thomas M. Skovholt
- Burnout: The Cost of Caring by Christina Maslach
- The Truth About Burnout: How Organizations Cause Personal Stress and What To Do About It by Christina Maslach and Michael P. Leiter
- Coping with Faculty Stress (Survival Skills for Scholars) by Walter H. Gmelch

Websites

- Burnout Self-Test (http://www.mindtools.com/pages/article/newTCS_08.htm)
- Job Burnout: Understand Symptoms and Take Action (http://www.mayoclinic.com/health/burnout/WL00062)

Podcasts

- Dear Dyslexic podcast Show: Episode 52 Dyslexia and Workplace Law with Barrister Ben Fogarty
- Dyslexic stories with Barrister Ben Fogarty Disability Discrimination and the law
- https://youtu.be/jd99EeVDUHk?si=biMiepnjNkC8j41Z

PSYCHOSOCIAL HAZARDS CHECKLIST FOR NEURODIVERGENT EMPLOYEES

Feedback Mechanisms:	Yes/No	Comments	Actions
Is there a feedback mechanism for employees to provide input on neurodiversity initiatives?			
Is feedback actively sought and used to improve neurodiversity programs and accommodations?			
Are regular assessments conducted to ensure the effectiveness of support systems for neurodivergent employees?			
Awareness and understanding:	**Yes/No**	**Comments**	**Actions**
Are employees and managers educated about different neurodivergent conditions?			

	Yes/No	Comments	Actions
Is there awareness about common challenges faced by neurodivergent individuals in the workplace?			
Are there training programs in place to foster understanding and inclusion?			
Communication	**Yes/No**	**Comments**	**Actions**
Is communication within the organisation diverse and accessible, accommodating different communication styles?			
Are there clear channels for employees to disclose neurodivergent conditions and request accommodations?			
Is there an open dialogue about neurodiversity, reducing stigma and fostering a supportive culture?			

Accommodations	Yes/No	Comments	Actions
Are reasonable accommodations provided for neurodivergent individuals, such as flexible work hours, quiet workspaces, or assistive technologies?			
Is there a formal process for requesting and implementing accommodation?			
Are managers and colleagues aware of and supportive in implementing accommodation?			
Work Environment	**Yes/No**	**Comments**	**Actions**
Is the physical workspace designed to minimise sensory overload, considering factors like lighting, noise levels and seating arrangements?			

	Yes/No	Comments	Actions
Are there quiet spaces available for employees who may need a break from sensory stimuli?			
Is the workplace structured to allow for flexibility in work styles and routines?			
Social Interaction	**Yes/No**	**Comments**	**Actions**
Are social interactions inclusive and considerate of different social styles?			
Is there training to promote understanding of social cues and communication preferences among neurodivergent individuals?			
Are team-building activities designed to be inclusive and accommodating e.g. group work doesn't include public reading and writing?			

Pre-readings provided prior to team events and training			
Performance Expectations	**Yes/No**	**Comments**	**Actions**
Are performance expectations communicated clearly, considering potential challenges for neurodivergent individuals?			
Is there flexibility in performance evaluations to account for diverse learning and working styles?			
Are managers trained to provide constructive feedback that considers neurodivergent perspectives using neuro-affirming language?			
Anti-Discrimination Policies:	**Yes/No**	**Comments**	**Actions**
Are there explicit anti-discrimination policies that encompass neurodivergence?			

Is there a clear process for reporting discrimination or harassment related to neurodivergence?			
Are employees educated about their rights and protections under these policies?			
Support Networks	**Yes/No**	**Comments**	**Actions**
Are there support networks or affinity groups for neurodivergent individuals within the organisation?			
Is there a designated point of contact or resources for employees seeking guidance or support, related to neurodivergence?			
Leadership Commitment:	**Yes/No**	**Comments**	**Actions**
Is there a visible commitment from organisational leadership to neurodiversity and inclusion?			

Are neurodivergent individuals represented in leadership positions?			
Is there ongoing evaluation and improvement of neurodiversity initiatives within the organisation?			
Are neurodivergent leaders provided with training opportunities to support self-awareness of their neurodivergence and their leadership role?			

This checklist is intended to guide organisations in assessing and addressing potential psychosocial hazards related to neurodivergence in the workplace. Tailoring these considerations to specific organisational contexts and continuously adapting practices are essential for creating an inclusive and supportive environment for all employees.

Chapter 8

SETTING DYSLEXIC TALENT UP FOR SUCCESS IN THE WORKPLACE

"In the middle of difficulty lies opportunity."
Albert Einstein

This chapter is a fun and creative one for you. Thank goodness, you might be thinking. I know, as I write, it's been heavy reading/listening up until now. From here on, you can put into action all that you've learnt! As you work through this section, another long one, I know I hope you have time to reflect and think and, by the end, put some concrete strategies in place for either yourself as a dyslexic or as someone who works with dyslexics and other neurodivergences. This section will not just support dyslexic and neurodivergent employees but also support all your team members. However, before we start to look at workplace accommodations, we need to understand the roles the dyslexic employee, the manager, the leadership team, and the organisation have to play in supporting the implementation of workplace accommodations. Workplace accommodations must reflect the foundation of good workplace practice, adhere to laws and legislation and align with universal design principles.

As you work your way through, ponder what workplace accommodations are available in your organisation. Are they easily accessible? Are they buried deep within a policy or procedure? Or are they non-existent? In your workplace, do dyslexics rely on their manager's discretion to access workplace accommodations, as mentioned earlier, which you now know can be a substantial barrier to success, or do they sit within your People and Culture or DEI team? Are you worried about the cost? If so, don't be. There are cost-effective options available that support neurodivergent conditions, so don't worry, we have that covered. So, let's get cracking and look at the roles played in successfully implementing accommodations in the workplace.

8.1. THE ROLE OF THE DYSLEXIC EMPLOYEE

It is vital that a dyslexic employee is able to self-advocate. This leads us to the elephant in the room – not all dyslexic people can do this. Remember there are three dyslexic neurodivergent personas in your workplace; those who talk about it and will self-advocate, those who will not share their disability, and those who don't know they have a disability/are different (but they do know something is not right). In an ideal world, we won't need to self-advocate because the environment would be set up for all of us to thrive, but that is not the way the world works, especially in the workplace for those with dyslexia. The ability to communicate one's needs, preferences and rights effectively, can be challenging for various reasons, as we have already worked through. Despite these challenges, developing self-advocacy skills is important for us to succeed. When we can self-advocate, we can feel a sense of self-determination, allowing us to have greater control over our lives in and out of the workplace

I find as dyslexics we are consistently having to self-advocate for our needs. From our early experiences in school, it was our parents advocating for our needs, but as we got older, it became our responsibility. I have a saying in my presentations it's not our fault we are dyslexic, but it is our responsibility, yet when we have to self-advocate all of the time, which takes a significant amount of mental effort, it can be quite taxing ... and that putting it politely. It adds a layer of complexity to our already demanding lives. Building self-confidence is essential for effective self-advocacy, and it is important to recognise that self-confidence can be negatively affected during our early years and as we transition into adulthood and beyond. We should not underestimate the challenges that self-advocacy brings, as it can often be difficult, and sometimes it seems easier to be an ostrich and bury our heads in the sand. For example, during my time at a previous organisation, as I have mentioned, I was given the nickname *'Albie' by the Chief Operating Officer.* This name was a reference to my struggles with financial analysis on spreadsheets. It was not uncommon for him to call out to me in front of colleagues, saying things like, "Oh Albie, your numbers are all mixed up again," often eliciting laughter from my manager, another Executive. This experience was both embarrassing and humiliating, and for someone in a senior management position, I felt much shame. At that moment, I lacked the self-confidence to advocate for myself and address the disrespectful way I was being spoken to. I have never forgiven myself for not having the ability to shut it down, to make a stand. Still, the deep-seated feeling we have about ourselves that stems from childhood, that negative self-talk and feeling of inadequacy, never goes away, which is why we need to quash it before it ever rears its ugly head in adulthood.

Now, many dyslexics are having to self-advocate for their rights in the workplace, and this can cause them to feel psychologically unsafe. Dyslexic employees have to disclose multiple times to different people in order to obtain the accommodations needed to be successful employees. Ideally, workplaces would implement disclosure and accommodation policies so this does not have to happen; by establishing clear systems and processes, we can minimise the need for individual self-advocacy, allowing everyone to focus on their work more efficiently. Based on universal design principles, all employees would benefit from the ways managers, team leaders and organisational structure work towards and promote inclusiveness.

8.2. THE ROLE OF THE MANAGER AND LEADERSHIP TEAM

'...I got this new manager who I disclosed to – I disclosed to that president as well, he was one of the great people in the initial interview. Then had this new manager arrive, showed him one of these investor relations reports and that's when he became really aggressive and said, you know, this is the worst piece of writing I've ever seen, this is not for a CEO...'
Research participant

The roles of management, leadership, human resources, diversity, equity, and inclusion (DEI), workplace health and safety, information technology and finance are all critical when considering how to effectively support and develop employees with dyslexia and other neurodivergence. Initiatives require collaborative effort across the entire organisation. You may be curious about the reasons for this approach; we will address that shortly. First, let us examine the responsibilities of the management and leadership teams.

As a manager or leader, the responsibility of building high-performing teams while achieving business key performance indicators (KPIs) can often feel overwhelming. This role presents both challenges and rewards, reflecting the importance of your position. Supporting and understanding issues related to dyslexia, neurodivergence and disability is a critical part of your responsibilities, and it can be difficult to manage alongside other priorities. However, after reviewing this chapter, you will find that these concepts are more manageable than they may seem. With the right individuals from your operational departments, it is possible to cultivate a highly-skilled, high-performing team that prioritises psychological safety, ultimately benefiting everyone involved.

Let's look at the research. In addition to exploring the workplace experiences of dyslexic employees, my research also looked at the culture of workplaces from the perspective of employers and managers working with dyslexic employees. The purpose of this was to really understand just how challenging it is to support dyslexic employees. There is little international research on managing a diverse workforce, and none within the Australian context. Given the high percentage of people with dyslexia across the population [102, 153, 207, 277, 308], this was surprising. Whilst some management and support of individuals with dyslexia may need to be industry or role specific, my work identified some common underlying principles for inclusive workplace practices, that could be applied to all settings.

Currently, we know there is an absence of comprehensive policies and procedures to promote inclusivity for individuals with dyslexia in organisations. Instead, employers and managers tend to approach each situation on an ad hoc basis, resulting in a lack of preparedness and competency in handling such disclosures. Study participants reported an overall absence of awareness, understanding and training opportunities at the organisational level to manage and support employees with dyslexia. The absence of explicit and precise workplace policies and procedures further compounds this issue.

Interestingly, when employers and managers were sympathetic and understanding, their staff felt safe to disclose their dyslexia, leading to positive outcomes for the employee and their employer. While it was fortunate that the participants in this study had prior experience of dyslexia with family members and previous staff, this will not be the case for all managers. It is therefore likely that, without the right training and organisational supports, many managers could feel ill-equipped, overwhelmed and susceptible to inadvertent discrimination when working with dyslexic staff.

My work indicated that for some individuals, the impact of their dyslexia did not become apparent until their work performance dropped. This often arose from changes to job structure, such as the introduction of new work processes, management, groups, or equipment. This finding is also supported by work undertaken by Winters (2020) and De Beer et al (2014). Conversely, my findings also found that supportive performance reviews could encourage disclosure of dyslexia and lead to performance improvement, particularly when employers and managers felt able to implement reasonable adjustments for the dyslexic employee.

One of my most important findings was that education, training, and access to dyslexic resources were perceived to be crucial to ensure managers and employees possessed the knowledge needed to perform their duties in the workplace. Equally, education and training were considered essential for developing an understanding of workplace policies in relation to disabilities, reasonable adjustments and equal opportunity. A key enabler for supporting employees with dyslexia, is to ensure workplaces understand dyslexia as a disability and develop a comprehensive awareness of the needs, strengths and weaknesses of dyslexic employees. Furthermore, managers and leadership teams have a responsibility to adhere to and understand the legal demands specified in the DDA, equality laws and the Fair Work Act. Employers and organisations are in a unique and exciting position to be able to provide truly inclusive and diverse workplaces, by embracing those with dyslexia and harnessing the strengths and qualities they bring to the workplace.

8.3. THE ROLE OF THE ORGANISATION

As mentioned above, the functions of management, leadership, human resources, diversity, equity, and inclusion (DEI), workplace health and safety, information technology and finance all play a vital role in the effective support and development of employees with dyslexia and other neurodivergent conditions. This initiative necessitates a collaborative effort across the organisation and an understanding of each area's complimentary role. You may not have all these departments in your organisation, so reflect on your own workplace. Below is my recommendation, based on the work we have done with countless organisations, to help reduce the need for employees to self-advocate. This should all be integrated into your policies and procedures as outlined below.

- **Manager** – Work with HR/ P&C to facilitate workplace accommodations and organise workplace training.
- **HR or P&C**: Help facilitate conversations with finance and IT to ensure workplace accommodations are easily accessible and installed.
- **Finances**: Easy process to pay for workplace accommodations and support services without the need for individuals to have to self-advocate or justify expense. Manager should be signing off on this.
- **IT department**: Install and enable assistive technology and AI pro-

grams to be accessible and not blocked by firewalls.

- **Work Health and Safety:** Purchase the tools and workplace accommodations needed, if not being funded through JobAccess.
- **DEI:** Help to advocate for the needs of the dyslexic employee with manager and HR if needed.

Setting individuals with dyslexia up for success in the workplace requires cultivating an environment that provides the necessary support, enabling them to excel in their roles and contribute to the organisation's objectives. This strategy is founded on recognising and valuing diverse abilities, ensuring employees with dyslexia have equal opportunities to realise their full potential. It comes back to your organisation's values and the culture you want to create. The following are key aspects to consider when fostering success for not just dyslexic employees but your entire workforce.

Understanding and Awareness: It is essential for employers, managers and colleagues to possess a foundational understanding of dyslexia, its effects on individuals and the potential challenges faced by dyslexic employees. Increasing awareness can lead to enhanced empathy and more effective support.

Accommodations: Easily accessible accommodations, which we will cover next. Remember, under the Disability Discrimination Act, those with dyslexia and other learning disabilities are entitled to workplace accommodations that facilitate equitable participation in their job role.

Communication: Establish open and transparent communication channels with dyslexic employees, encouraging them to express their needs, preferences and concerns regarding their work responsibilities. Regular check-ins can help ensure they feel comfortable and excel in their roles.

Training and Resources: Implement training sessions for all employees to raise awareness of dyslexia and other neurodivergences, especially for managers, leadership and executives. Research tells us there is a significant lack of understanding and awareness, so training is a must. Training can guide how to foster an inclusive and supportive work environment. Ensure that resources, such as assistive technology tools and accessibility guidelines, are readily accessible.

Tailored Documented Support: Collaborate with dyslexic employees to develop documented personalised support plans. This can be in the style of a workplace accommodations passport or a workplace accommodation form. This may involve identifying and documenting strategies that are most effective for them, including specific software, modified communication methods or additional training. This also helps if their line manager leaves or they change positions in the organisation, and reduces the need for the employee to disclose to multiple departments. This document, with permission from the employee, can be utilised to share relevant information with IT, finance and HR, reducing the need for ongoing disclosure.

Accessible Materials: Ensure all written materials, documents and presentations are designed with accessibility in mind. Utilise clear fonts, appropriate formatting and concise
language to improve readability.

Inclusive Workspaces: Create workspaces that accommodate the needs of dyslexic employees. Consider factors such as lighting, noise levels and organisation, to establish an environment conducive to focus and productivity.

Feedback and Recognition: Provide constructive feedback and recognition to dyslexic employees for their contributions. Acknowledging their efforts and achievements enhances their confidence and motivation.

Career Development: Ensure dyslexic employees have access to opportunities for career development and advancement, including training, mentoring and skills enhancement. Resources that facilitate their growth within the organisation should be made available.

Advocacy and Support Groups: Research has found that establishing support groups or networks within the workplace, where dyslexic employees can connect, share experiences and provide mutual support, can be beneficial. This sense of community can offer invaluable emotional assistance and help with advocacy needs.

Allocated budget: Understand and tap into JobAccess funding and having an allocated budget to support dyslexic and other neurodivergent employees is essential to your success as an organisation. Through JobAccess you will get 1;1 support, workplace accommodations and training, all paid for by the Federal Government. There really is no excuse not to be providing training and workplace accommodations in your workplace. This funding enables you to allocate a budget for those employees who do not have a diagnosis but may be struggling. A great example is *The Digital Picnic* who pay for their employees to access diagnostic assessments. Amazing!

Policies and procedures: Integrate disability/neurodivergent workplace accommodations, processes and funding support into *business as usual* by including these in your policies and procedures, across the employment life cycle from recruitment through to career progression. It needs to be explicit so people feel safe to ask. We want to reduce the risk of passing and coping with dyslexic employees, we want to make them feel safe to ask for help, not hide in the shadows.

Fostering success for dyslexic employees necessitates a comprehensive approach that integrates awareness, accommodations, education and a supportive culture. When employers take proactive measures to create an inclusive workplace, dyslexic employees are empowered to thrive and make meaningful contributions to the organisation's success.

8.4. REFRAMING WORKPLACES USING UNIVERSAL DESIGN PRINCIPLES

Universal design principles encompass a set of guidelines designed to create environments, products and systems that are accessible to a diverse range of individuals, regardless of age, ability or other characteristics. The principles originated in architecture and are used now within the educational and higher education sectors to create more inclusive learning environments; an educational framework that guides the design of flexible learning environments and materials to accommodate individual learning differences. UDL principles aim to make learning accessible for all students.

These principles have now expanded across various domains, including workplaces, with the aim of promoting inclusivity and eliminating barriers. The seven principles, articulated by Connell et al. in 1997, cover aspects such as

- equitable use,
- flexibility in use
- simple and intuitive us
- perceptible information
- tolerance for error
- low physical effort
- size and space considerations for approach and use, as exampled below [288].

In the context of designing inclusive workplaces, the application of universal design principles is instrumental. These principles are used in educational settings and that look at ways to accommodate all individuals, recognising and addressing variations in abilities, preferences and needs. This inclusivity is not limited to employees with disabilities, it extends to all employees to meet the varying needs and working styles. By eliminating physical and communication barriers, universal design ensures that workspaces, technology and information are accessible to everyone, promoting equal opportunities and participation in work-related tasks [284, 288].

Moreover, workplaces designed with universal principles contribute to enhanced productivity. Examples of universal design principles for the workplace include editing software like Grammarly on everyone's computer, access to quiet rooms, and everyone has the option to use noise-cancelling headphones, dimmable lights and flexible working arrangements. These are all universal design principles that benefit the whole organisation.

Okay, so when you are thinking about workplace accommodations, don't just think about them from a dyslexic employee perspective, but think about how you could use them more broadly to support your team and workplace.

8.5. WHAT ARE WORKPLACE ACCOMMODATIONS?

Workplace adjustments refer to modifications made to a workplace or work process to accommodate the needs of an individual with a disability or medical condition. These adjustments can help create a more accessible and inclusive workplace for all employees, including those with dyslexia. For dyslexics, workplace adjustments can come in a variety of forms; it's not just about better access to assistive technology, although AI really is our best friend! Many accommodations are also at little or no additional financial cost and may just mean adjusting your current work practices. Often when adjusting current work practice, many changes will benefit all staff.

We know that internal workplace policies around workplace accommodations are not sufficient to support employees with dyslexia and other neurodivergence. They are broad and reflect disabilities in general terms, rather than specifically neurodivergence. This is despite the attempts of policy and legislation to increase the participation of workers with disabilities [116, 120, 121]. In workplaces where employees fear discrimination and stigma, they are forced to execute their own strategies to manage and keep up with workplace demands, and this can lead to mental exhaustion, stress and anxiety. Yes, we have covered this point already, but just so you don't forget - workplaces must develop an understanding about what constitutes a 'reasonable adjustment' to provide appropriate support to employees with dyslexia. You might be thinking, *What? I need policies and procedures on neurodivergence now?* Well, yes. But instead of having exclusive policies and procedures on neurodivergence, consider how you could embed this into current policies and procedures.

Here are some workplace accommodations that are helpful to those with dyslexia, other neurodivergence and your staff, more broadly. With technology and AI moving so fast, by the time this book goes to print there will be new tools available, but it's not all about tech and AI, and I am sure you will already be using some of these:

8.6. ASSISTIVE TECHNOLOGY

Access to assistive technology is a game changer, and we cannot succeed without access to assistive technology -; it's a must-have, not a nice-to-have! This could include text-to-speech software, screen readers, spell-checking software and speech recognition software. Don't let your IT department become the barrier; we need them to be the enabler. Many times, I have undertaken hours of work with a dyslexic employee, only to find their IT department won't allow them to use the software we find is most helpful, leaving everyone feeling disappointed and let down. We will speak about this further in this chapter. Here are several ways technology can assist dyslexics in the workplace:

- **Text-to-Speech Software**: Dyslexic individuals often struggle with reading and comprehending written text. Text-to-speech software can help by converting written content into spoken words, making it easier for them to understand and process information.
- **Speech-to-Text Software**: Dyslexics may find it easier to express their ideas verbally rather than in writing. Speech-to-text software allows them to dictate their thoughts, which can then be converted into written text. This can be particularly useful for writing emails, reports or other documents.
- **Word Prediction and Autocorrect**: Word prediction software suggests words as a user types, which can help dyslexics by reducing the need to remember complex spelling. Autocorrect can catch and correct spelling errors, making written communication more accurate.
- **Customisable Fonts and Backgrounds**: Some people find certain fonts and background colours more readable than others. This can easily be done through Microsoft Immersion. Customisable settings in digital devices and applications allow users to adjust text appearance to suit their preferences. For me personally, I like extra-large font and double spacing.
- **Digital Note-Taking Tools**: Digital note-taking apps allow dyslexic individuals to organise their thoughts more effectively. They can use features like voice recordings, typed notes, and images to create comprehensive records of meetings and tasks. These tools can be super helpful to use during meetings if you are a minute-taker or you need to make important notes for a meeting. Many of the cli-

ents I work with use *Remarkable Note Pad*. This is just one example.

- **Organisational Apps**: Some people might benefit from apps designed to help with time management, task scheduling and organisation. Visual reminders and easy-to-use interfaces can make managing tasks and responsibilities less overwhelming. I find Trello is a great tool for organisation workflow and for keeping notes of different tasks.

- **Mind Mapping and Visual Diagrams**: Visual thinking tools like mind-mapping software can assist dyslexics in brainstorming, planning projects and understanding complex concepts by using visual diagrams. I have a giant whiteboard that has all my ideas and plans mapped out. I also like to draw when I am explaining concepts or ideas. Granted they are usually stick figures, but it gets the message across!

- **E-books, Audiobooks and Podcasts**: For many, traditional reading can be challenging. E-books and audiobooks provide alternative ways to access information. Many workplace materials and resources are available in digital formats. This is one of my favourite ways to learn new information. I put my ear buds in and off I go for a walk. It's a great why to unwind at the end of the day before I pick up my daughter, while getting some exercise in.

- **Learning Management Systems (LMS)**: If training or professional development is necessary, dyslexic employees can benefit from learning platforms that offer multimedia content, interactive modules and alternative formats for learning materials.

- **Accessibility Features**: Modern operating systems and software often include accessibility features specifically designed to support users with dyslexia. These features might include magnification, screen readers, and colour contrast adjustments.

- **Proofreading and Grammar Checking Software**: All those with dyslexia will be using some type of spell checker, but if we are talking universal design, then let's look at tools that the whole workplace can use, such as Grammarly; a tool everyone can benefit from.

- **Virtual Assistants**: Voice-activated virtual assistants can help dyslexics with a variety of tasks, from setting reminders and sending messages to searching for information on the internet.

It's important to note that individual preferences and needs vary, so it's a good idea for dyslexic individuals to explore different technologies and find the ones that work best for them. Additionally, employers can create an inclusive environment by offering support, understanding, and access to the necessary tools for employees with dyslexia. As an employer you need to be open to your staff accessing this type of technology and, at times, your IT security needs to be assessed to ensure your dyslexic staff can use the tools needed to do their work. It's extremely frustrating when I go into workplaces and conduct a learning and development planning session with a dyslexic employee to find out their IT department won't allow the software needed to perform their job. It's very disheartening for the dyslexic individual.

8.7. NON-TECH SUPPORT

There are lots of free non-tech solutions out there. You are probably already using some of them, but let's take a look now. Remember these strategies will not just support dyslexics to work at their best but also your teams and workplace as a whole.

Providing Materials Early: Distributing agendas, documents, reports and reading materials well in advance of meetings allows employees with dyslexia to process the information at their own pace. This is crucial for complex topics, enabling dyslexics to prepare adequately, reducing anxiety and improving participation.

Clear Formatting: Clear and accessible formatting can aid comprehension and reading of documents. This includes using larger fonts, bullet points, bolding key points, using colour, though not red or yellow, avoiding dense blocks of text and the use of all capitals. I tell people if it's more than a paragraph in an email, I won't read it. It just takes me too long to process and I have to go back over it many times.

Allowing Extra Time: This is critical, and like the assistive tech for completing tasks or projects, enabling extra time can significantly alleviate pressure; this allows employees to engage with the material thoroughly, leading to more thoughtful and accurate outputs and engagement. Dyslexics require additional time to complete tasks that involve reading and writing, as we have already discussed. This is a cost-free adjustment too!

Verbal Feedback: Encouraging verbal feedback rather than immediate written responses, can help employees articulate their thoughts more clearly. This approach recognises the processing challenges that may arise when reading and writing under time constraints. My supervisors would always ask me to record my verbal explanations and then translate them into my writing because my verbal skills are so much stronger than my writing skills. Having the dyslexic record the verbal explanation might help them when they are then transiting it into text.

Taking Questions on Notice: It should be acceptable for employees to take questions on notice if they cannot provide an immediate answer. This practice not only respects their processing needs but also fosters a culture of thoughtful engagement rather than rushed responses.

Flexible working hours: Some people with dyslexia may feel cognitive overload and mental fatigue by the end of the day, so enabling flexible working hours can support them to work to the best of their ability. While flexible working hours are also great for those who are carers/parents and since COVID, it really this has become *business as* *usual* for most, if not all workplaces, however it is still a good reminder.

Providing instructions in a dyslexia-friendly format: Employers can provide verbal instructions in follow-up written or a dyslexia-friendly format, audio files and videos. If you need to provide written instructions, use bullet points avoid lengthy emails, and I find larger-spaced fonts to be helpful.

Providing support and training: Employers need to provide training on dyslexia awareness and accommodations for all employees, especially HR and leadership. It is also helpful to have dyslexic/neurodivergent training can provide dyslexics with support and training, including coaching, mentoring and access to dyslexia support groups. This will be further explored below. Workplace training for non-dyslexic employees is a must and we will discuss that later in this chapter.

8.8. THE ROLE OF MENTORS AND COACHING EMPLOYEES WITH DYSLEXIA

As we have just discussed, it's not all about technology when it comes to workplace accommodations and support. One of the most valuable supports for a dyslexic person can be a mentor, coach, and/or peer support. Again, this is not something that is just good for dyslexics; everyone can benefit from a mentor, coach and/or peer support. There are numerous benefits in having external people who you can debrief too, including a psychologist and or counsellor, which I strongly advocate for, This can help with self-reflection and the sharing of ideas and thoughts.

A mentor and coach can play important roles in supporting dyslexic employees, helping them to succeed in the workplace. There is a substantial amount of research looking at the role of mentors, coaches and peer support in other neurodivergent cohorts, which can be applicable to dyslexics as well. My research found that when managers paired up a dyslexic employee with a non-dyslexic employee, the magic happened because they were working to their strengths. Let's unpack this now.

8.1 Mentoring and peer support

A mentor is typically someone who has more experience and expertise in a particular field or industry than the mentee. The role of a mentor for a dyslexic employee is to provide guidance, advice and support based on their own lived experiences. This can include providing career advice, helping the dyslexic employee navigate workplace challenges offering feedback on their performance and looking at strengths and areas of difficulty,

Mentorship by another dyslexic or neurodivergent can be especially important as it can provide a supportive relationship with someone who understands their unique challenges and can help them navigate those challenges in the workplace. I currently have a dyslexic mentor for the first time, and it has been really helpful to have someone who really understands the challenges we can face. It can be really isolating at times, particularly in the workplace, or if you have just been diagnosed and you don't really know any other people who are dyslexic. A mentor to work things through can reduce feelings of isolation and help with managing the stress and anxiety that can often accompany workplace challenges. They can also support with self-advocacy needs, such as workplace accommodations. If you are unable to find a dyslexic mentor, then connecting with other employees with disabilities can be helpful, especially if there is a disability or neurodivergent network within your workplace. You can also join a dyslexic Facebook group or contact us at rethinkdyslexia.com.au, and we can see how we can help.

8.2 Learning and development support through coaching

A coach, in contrast, primarily focuses on assisting dyslexic employees to develop and work on specific skills and reach designated goals. The coaching process facilitates individuals' identification of their strengths and weaknesses, clarification of their objectives, creation of action plans, and overcoming challenges to achieve desired outcomes. It aims to inspire hope and motivation, reinforcing individuals' confidence in their ability to surmount obstacles and foster a positive mindset [317], as well as help identify any resources or support they may need to achieve their goal.

At re:think dyslexia, we see a variety of clients through our learning and development coaching program. We currently work with dyslexics, ADHDers, autistic and AudHDers (Autistic/ADHDers). The majority of our clients are women, with a late diagnosis. From a dyslexic perspective, our coaching emphasises both personal and professional development. Here are some ways the coaching we deliver through re:think dyslexia, helps those with dyslexia and other neurodivergence:

Some of the areas we work on include:
Clarify goals: Coaching can help individuals to identify and clarify their goals, which can be especially important for individuals with dyslexia, who may struggle with organisation and time management.

Develop action plans: Coaching can help individuals develop specific, actionable plans for achieving their goals. This can help them stay focused and motivated, break larger goals into smaller, more manageable steps, and stay accountable.

Build self-awareness: Coaching can help build self-awareness and identify strengths and weaknesses, especially if the client has recently been diagnosed. It can also help map out what workplace accommodations are needed to support specific workplace challenges the client is facing.

Build confidence: Coaching can help individuals build confidence and self-efficacy, which can be especially important for dyslexics who may have experienced negative feedback or criticism in the past. This also helps build self-advocacy skills needed to navigate workplaces.

Overall, mentors and coaching are valuable tools that can multiple benefits for dyslexics to thrive in the workplace.

8.9. AUSTRALIAN FUNDING SUPPORT

Did you know that funding support is available for individuals who are neurodivergent, including those with learning disabilities such as dyslexia, dysgraphia, dyspraxia, and dyscalculia, as well as ADHD and autism? Currently, learning disabilities and ADHD are not included in the NDIS, and it seems unlikely that learning disabilities will ever be covered under NDIS. As a result, dyslexics, especially children, are facing challenges in accessing appropriate support compared to other neuro-developmental groups.

Funding is available in Australia through JobAccess, which operates under the Employment Assistance Fund. For many adults with dyslexia, it may not be necessary to be enrolled in the NDIS, as Job-Access provides valuable support. However, we recognise that many individuals with dyslexia are not performing at the level appropriate with their training and educational background, and this is where Job-Access can play a significant role in addressing this problem. This initiative allows neurodivergent employees to access one-on-one support and workplace accommodations, at no cost to them or their employer, while also providing employers with free workplace training. Many clients I have worked with, have expressed sincere relief and gratitude upon learning about the financial assistance available to them through JobAccess. This support is particularly significant for individuals with dyslexia, who have historically faced difficulties in obtaining funding. Let's take a look at these programs in more detail now.

8.9.1. What is the Employment Assistance Fund

Employment Assistance Fund is an Australian Government initiative that aims to provide financial help to eligible people with disability and mental health conditions, as well as employers, to buy work-related modifications, equipment and workplace assistance and support services. The EAF is available to eligible people with disability, who are about to start a job, are self-employed or are currently working.

8.9.2. What is JobAccess?

JobAccess is an Australian Government initiative that offers support and resources to individuals with disabilities and those who employ them. It is aimed at facilitating access to employment opportunities. Acting under the Employment Assistance Fund (EAF), its primary objective is to assist people with disabilities, injuries or health conditions in finding and sustaining meaningful employment.

JobAccess provides various services to support individuals with disabilities in the workplace, including advice and information on workplace adjustments, available funding, and other relevant support services.

Benefits to employees, those who are self-employed and or seeking employment:

- Workplace Modifications: Providing financial assistance for necessary equipment, changes in the work environment.
- Access to specialised services to enable employees with disabilities to effectively perform their job responsibilities, such as one-to-one coaching and learning and development support.

Benefits for Employers

- Providing guidance on the hiring and retention of employees with disabilities.
- Offering financial assistance for workplace modifications
- specialised support services
- Disability/neurodivergent workplace training.

This is a reimbursement scheme, for a nominal fee, to cover the above-mentioned workplace accommodations, specialised services and training, so it's all free ... can you believe that? Reflecting on my own experiences, I believe that having access to one-on-one support sessions with someone who understands dyslexia could have been transformative during my formative years, and I see similar positive impacts on the individuals we assist today.

8.10. MENTAL HEALTH SUPPORT IN THE WORKPLACE

We have touched on the co-occurring mental health challenges those with dyslexia can face. Many organisations run a variety of mental health and well-being programs, from yoga to walking groups, 10,000-step challenges and access to psychologists and counsellors. One example is the Employment Assistance Program (EAP), different from the above-mentioned EAP, which is offered by many organisations and aims to provide free mental health support to their employees who may be struggling in or out of the workplace. The Employment Assistance Program is designed to provide confidential mental health support to employees, recognising that mental well-being is integral to job performance and satisfaction. Key features of this program include:

- **Free Access to Services for employees**: Employers fund the program, allowing employees to access mental health support without financial barriers. **Confidentiality:** The services provided are confidential, encouraging employees to seek help without fear of stigma or repercussions.

- **Comprehensive Support:** The program may include counselling, coaching, and psychologists. It aims to build coping strategies, enhance resilience, and improve overall mental health. By addressing mental health proactively, organisations are helping their employees manage their mental health challenges more effectively.

The positive impact of mental health support through programs like the Employment Assistance Program cannot be overstated. By providing employees with the tools and resources they need to manage their mental health, organisations can enhance job performance, reduce absenteeism and foster a supportive workplace culture. Many of those who participated in my research, as well as through my work, have accessed EAP services and it has been especially helpful in reducing the financial barrier of accessing these services, along with the barrier of timely support. In Australia, it can be difficult to have access to timely mental health support, and EAP is a great example of readily available workplace mental health support.

However, what we have found, is that some neurodivergent employees feel the general EAP services can lack the skills and knowledge to support neurodivergence and the intersectionality of mental health, workplace challenges and their disability/difference. That is why we have created the Neurodivergent Employment Assistance Program. It addresses the co-occurring mental health challenges, faced by individuals with dyslexia, and highlights the need for comprehensive support systems in the workplace. The NEAP serves as a vital resource, offering free and confidential mental health support to employees. By addressing mental health proactively and linking to JobAccess, organisations can not only improve the well-being of their employees, but also create a more inclusive and productive work environment. This expansion emphasises the importance of mental health support for individuals with dyslexia, particularly in the context of the Employment Assistance Program, and illustrates how such initiatives can positively influence both employee well-being and organisational outcomes.

8.11. CONCLUSION
This chapter offers practical guidance for implementing what you've learned so far, particularly in supporting dyslexic and neurodivergent employees in the workplace. It covers the importance of workplace accommodations, emphasising that these adjustments benefit not just dyslexic individuals but the entire team. The chapter also stresses the need for self-advocacy, recognising that many dyslexic employees may struggle to assert their needs due to past experiences and a lack of confidence.

Key points include the role of employers, managers and workplace culture, in fostering an inclusive environment. The absence of comprehensive policies often leads to ad hoc management of dyslexia, which can result in unintentional discrimination. Education, training and awareness are crucial in equipping employers and employees to handle dyslexia effectively.

The chapter also highlights universal design principles as a way to create inclusive workplaces that accommodate diverse needs. It explores various workplace accommodations, both technological (e.g., assistive software) and non-technological (e.g., flexible working hours). Additionally, the chapter underscores the value of mentoring, coaching and peer support in helping dyslexic employees succeed.

Finally, it touches on Australian funding support for neurodivergent employees, particularly through JobAccess, which offers financial assistance for workplace modifications and training. Mental health support is also discussed, with a focus on the Employment Assistance Program (EAP) and the need for specialised services that understand the unique challenges of neurodivergent individuals.

Overall, the chapter emphasises a holistic approach to supporting dyslexic employees, advocating for a combination of awareness, accommodations and a supportive workplace culture.

KEY TAKE-HOME MESSAGES

Workplace Accommodations Benefit Everyone: Adjustments made to support dyslexic and neurodivergent employees, such as assistive technology and flexible work arrangements, often improve the work environment for all team members.

Self-Advocacy is Essential but Challenging: Dyslexic employees need to develop self-advocacy skills to communicate their needs effectively. However, this can be difficult due to past experiences and a lack of confidence.

Inclusive Workplaces Require Comprehensive Policies: The absence of clear policies and training on managing dyslexia can lead to ad hoc and potentially discriminatory practices. Organisations should develop and implement comprehensive policies to support neurodivergent employees.

Universal Design Principles Foster Inclusivity: Applying universal design principles in the workplace helps create an environment that is accessible to all employees, not just those with disabilities.

Mentorship and Coaching are Vital: Providing dyslexic employees with mentors, coaches and peer support can significantly enhance their success and well-being in the workplace.

Funding Support is Available: In Australia, JobAccess provides financial assistance for workplace modifications and specialised support for neurodivergent employees, making it easier for them and their employers to access necessary resources.

Mental Health Support is Crucial: Programs like the Employment Assistance Program (EAP) are essential for providing confidential mental health support to employees, including those with dyslexia, helping to foster a more inclusive and supportive workplace culture.

Holistic Approach is Key: Supporting dyslexic employees requires a combination of awareness, appropriate accommodations and a culture that values and understands diverse abilities.

CASE STUDY 1: MAYA AND JOBACCESS

Maya, a team leader in an organisation of 300 employees, was diagnosed with dyslexia at the age of thirty-five. In her role, which she has held for three months, she manages a team of thirty staff members and has been aware of her condition for six months. To proactively address her needs, Maya sought dyslexia coaching prior to assuming her current position.

After two months in her role, she recognised the necessity for additional support, leading her to disclose her dyslexia to her team and request adjustments in their communication style. Maya also approached her manager to discuss accessing JobAccess for one-on-one support and workplace training, as recommended by her dyslexia learning and development coach. Following this, Maya and her manager coordinated with Human Resources, resulting in approval for Maya to apply for funding through JobAccess. With assistance from her coach, Maya completed the application process for one-on-one support and a workplace training session with JobAccess. On approval from JobAccess, Maya commenced her 1:1 sessions with her dyslexia learning and development coach.

After successfully finishing her support sessions, she was required to disclose her dyslexia to the IT department regarding the AI accommodations identified as beneficial for her role. Unfortunately, this process was lengthy, taking over two months for security checks, during which the urgency of her request was not prioritised, resulting in Maya struggling with her workload.

During this time, Maya also organised dyslexia awareness training in collaboration with the Diversity, Equity and Inclusion (DEI) team, which necessitated additional disclosure of her condition. Ultimately, she needed to arrange for funds to be reimbursed by JobAccess back to her cost centre, making this the fifth occasion she disclosed her disability. The cumulative effect of advocating for her support needs, while managing her regular responsibilities left Maya feeling overwhelmed and psychologically unsafe, due to the repeated necessity of discussing her condition

Questions

1. Reflecting on what you have learnt in this chapter, what could you do differently in your organisation to reduce the need for this to occur for employees like Maya?
2. How could you create a more psychologically safe environment for her?

RESOURCES

There are a huge number of resources you can find, so we are listing just a few to help you on your journey of discovery and understanding. You can find more information at re:think dyslexia.com.au. If you found any of this content distressing, please seek support:

- Lifeline on 13 11 14
- Beyond Blue - counsellor on 1300 22 4636
- NEAP Neurodivergent Employment Assistance Program on 1800 13 6327

Organisations supporting neurodivergent adults:

- re:think dyslexia
- JobAccess
- ADHD Australia

Books, podcasts, websites, support and more

- Work by Nancy Doyle and Almuth McDowall
- Neurodiversity Coaching: A Psychological Approach to Supporting Neurodivergent Talent and Career Potential
- Websites
- Centre for Excellence in Universal Design
- JobAccess Workplace Accommodations: Disability and Adjustment
- Human Rights Commission: Reasonable adjustment

Chapter 9
LOOKING AFTER YOURSELF AS A DYSLEXIC ADULT

Piglet, there is nothing in this
world that can HURT
you as much
as your own thoughts

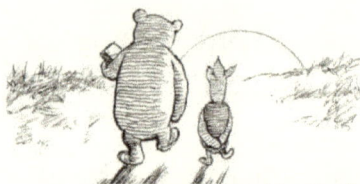

But Pooh, there's nothing in this
world that can HEAL
you as much
as your own thoughts

Winne-the-Pooh [1]

This is a short chapter before we wrap up what has been an epic journey
of learning and discovery, but it would be remiss of me not to take this

opportunity to outline some strategies I have learnt myself and through my work, that can support you, my fellow dyslexic, who is reading or listening to this book. These thoughts draw on my research, my own lived-experiences and the lived-experiences of young people and adults with dyslexia and other neurodivergences, who I have crossed paths with through my work with **re:think dyslexia** and the Dear Dyslexic Foundation. I started this work in 2015; I began with podcasts to share stories of other adults like me who felt lost, isolated and alone; and it has grown to be an internationally listened to podcast. Over the years of working with dyslexics and in my research, what has been apparent, is the sheer determination, resilience and perseverance of my fellow community members. So, how do we draw on our strengths to help us with our self-care?

The biggest lessons I have learnt have been around getting to understand myself and my difficulties, the importance of self-care and accepting who I am. We all know exercise and eating healthy are major protective factors to our self-care, but what does self-care look like for you?

What I learned, is the need for us to find ways that brings us joy, that help us feel connected and to feel good about ourselves. That right to feel good about ourselves was taken away from many of us at a young age, whether it was through education trauma, being humiliated, laughed at, misunderstood, name calling, feelings of being incompetent and the inability to fit in, to be *normal!* The list goes on, and this is supposed to be an uplifting chapter! A lot was taken away from many of us as children; the ability to really understand what was happening for us, the opportunity to access a diagnosis and early intervention, the chance to obtain an education and attain a job that we are highly capable of doing. Then, there is the inability to get a job that we are trained for. There is a lot of grief that comes with diagnosis of dyslexia/learning disabilities and for those who are not diagnosed until adulthood, I believe that grief is bigger. The baggage and scars I carry are deep seated, and no one will ever really understand those scars. They will never understand the daily challenges we face, that are so easy for others to do. But first, we must find ways to look after ourselves and there are many ways to do that. I wanted this to be a reminder to find something you love that re-energises you, helps to reduce the cognitive overload and helps you to build your self-esteem and confidence. So, I will share with you what helps me on a good day, and others as well. Self-care comes in many forms. Working on research and helping other dyslexics, for me, is self-care. Through my own experiences and those who I work with, as well as what the research is telling us, here is a list of different ways we can look at self-care that may be helpful for you:

Engage in Activities You Enjoy
When my mum was dying, I threw myself into my research; it was my safe space to go where I could shut out the noise, the pain, the grief. I also found getting outside with my daughter and playing music together, where we sing and dance, to be very helpful. Balance work and responsibilities with hobbies or activities that bring you joy and relaxation. Creative outlets, such as art, music or writing, can be particularly therapeutic. I love working in the garden when I have spare time. I love growing my own vegetables and it helps me feel closer to my mum, as she loved gardening too. I also love a good glass of wine or gin with a delicious cheese platter - now for me, that is a great way to unwind and enjoy time with my friends and family.

Prioritise Mental Health
Tigger who leant this from Budda was right, *'there is nothing in this world that can heal you as much as your own thoughts .'* Which is why

looking after and prioritising our mental health and well-being is so important. If we don't, our difficulties, baggage and trauma can all affect our relationships, our work and what we think and feel about ourselves. I know if I'm overwhelmed, tired or frustrated I can really have difficulties regulating my emotions, especially if I'm in an argument with my husband. My words get confused, my brain goes into overload, and I cannot articulate myself.

The risk of burnout is high. There is no research on dyslexic burnout but like autistic burnout, I believe dyslexic burnout does exist, we have seen how it can play out in the workplace. We need research into the impact of dyslexic burnout. If you have listened to my podcasts, you will know how much I advocate for a psychologist and/or mental health support; a mentor or a coach. It is so important to have sounding board, an objective person to talk through the ups and downs of life and to proactively take care of our mental health. If we are not proactive, things get hard. Having the self-awareness to put these strategies in place is so important as we try to manage our difficulties with life - because life can be hard.

Practice relaxation techniques, such as deep breathing, yoga or progressive muscle relaxation in your daily routine. Other activities I like to do, include meditation, not mediation. (I once sent a weekly calendar invite out to the whole organisation asking them to join me for mediation, when it was supposed to be meditation!)

Mindfulness apps are really a great help, especially when feeling overwhelmed. I have tried journal writing but as someone with dysgraphia, I find the activity quite hard and not as enjoyable, but it might work for you. Regular physical activity can also help manage stress and improve overall well-being.

SLEEP!!!

Sleep is my favourite pastime. I have always been a napper, and

I could have an afternoon sleep anywhere, at any time. It has always been a source of amusement for my family and friends. I have come to realise, over time, this has been a way for me to manage my neurodivergence. It is the only time my brain stops; it's like I have car engine running in my head non-stop and it was only recently I learnt that this is not *normal*. Having a toddler has reduced my ability to nap, which is quite distressing, so now I go to bed early to compensate for no naps.

Practice Self-Compassion

Understanding ourselves, our condition and what we need, is really important to help us be proactive in managing work, family and the day-today challenges that life brings us - because as we all know, there are many. We need to find what our strengths are and draw on them, whenever we can, to help mitigate those feelings of *not being good enough*. Acknowledge your efforts and accomplishments, no matter how small. Avoid negative self-talk. Remind yourself that dyslexia is just one aspect of who you are.

Create a Supportive Environment

Surround yourself with understanding and supportive people, both personally and professionally. Seek out mentors, coaches or peer support groups who can relate to your experiences. We have built a community over the last eight years from the Dear Dyslexic Podcast show; the Dear Dyslexic Facebook group is creating an Australia community for young people and adults. There are lots of overseas groups you can find as well, that can be helpful.

Reducing cognitive overload

Having quiet, where there is no sound except for my overworked computer battery and the sound of the wind outside. I find that *quiet* really helps me to stay calm and to not feel overwhelmed. Too much noise and I feel like my brain is going into meltdown and I can't cope. Sometimes I have to say to my family, 'I can't cope,' and need to step away when there is too much happening.

Develop a Routine
This can be hard especially if you are dyslexic/ADHD. No matter how many times I have tried to create routines, write lists, buy multiple planners and organisers, I just can't stick to it. My mind is all over the place. Actually, the lists do help to calm my mind at night, sometimes. But if you can establish daily routines that include time for work, rest and relaxation, and use planners, apps or visual aids to help manage your schedule and stay organised, you may feel more in control and have less cognitive overload.

Utilise Assistive Technology
Another way to reduce cognitive overload is to use the tools! It is hard when we are stuck in our old ways of doing things and changing habits takes time, but honestly, I couldn't live without AI tools now. I need less human support with my writing and editing and I am much more efficient with my work and time management. Leverage tools like text-to-speech, speech-to-text and organisational apps to reduce cognitive load and improve efficiency, as we discussed earlier. I promise you, these tools will change your life for the better ... FOREVER.

Allow Extra Time and setting achievable goals
I am always late, no matter how much time I think I have; I actually don't have enough. In the ADHD world, they call this time blindness. I think I have enough time, so I will put out the washing, unpack the dishwasher, oh and make a coffee ... and then I'm fifteen minutes

late. We need more time to do most things, so give it to yourself. Give yourself additional time to complete reading, writing or any task that requires more cognitive effort for you to be organised, or just on time. Avoid rushing, which can increase stress and reduce the quality of your work. Set achievable goals that align with your strengths and interests. Avoid setting overly high expectations that can lead to frustration or burnout.

Advocate for Your Needs
Unfortunately, we are always having to self-advocate for our needs. I feel as I get older, it's easier because I just don't care what people think anymore. But this has taken time and as I have watched the autistic community, who are so good at it, I feel I, and us as a community, should be able to as well. I know there seems to be a lot more support and awareness for the autistic community, but our time is coming and there is lots we can learn from them.

If we don't advocate for our needs at home, school and work, we will not be working to the best of our ability. This includes educating ourselves about what's out there. Stay informed about dyslexia and neurodiversity to better understand your strengths and challenges. Share your knowledge with others to foster a more supportive environment at work or home.

Reach out to our community or me at **re:think dyslexia** if you are needing some help.

Don't hesitate to request accommodations that can make tasks easier for you.

Build a Positive Work-Life Balance
Ensure that your work does not consume all your time and energy; make space for relaxation, hobbies and social connections. Set bound-

aries to protect your personal time and prevent burnout. Ask for help
if you need it; if you can't speak to your workplace or your family, then
connect with us.

Stay Connected with Your Values
Regularly reflect on what matters most to you and align your activities and goals with those values. Let your values guide your decisions,
reducing the stress that can come from trying to meet external expectations.

These are just some self-care strategies I could think of that might
be able to help you manage day-to-day more effectively while reducing
the risk of dyslexic burnout and fostering a sense of well-being and
empowerment. In a world of work, where we are constantly having
to adjust ourselves to cope with the environment around us and for
people to understand us, cognitive overload and mental fatigue are real.
While the world continues to not understand us, we have to ensure we
are looking after ourselves, and you don't have to go it alone - there is a
community here to help and support us in any way it can.

Chapter 10

THE DYSLEXIC GOLDEN THREADS THAT CREATE THE TAPESTRY OF LIFE

Doing nothing encourages the status quo. We must make a conscious decision to reject the status quo to improve the quality-of-life outcomes for those with dyslexia, their families, and the broader community.
Dr Shae Wissell

Oh my gosh, you made it and what a journey we've had. The hard part is over. You have stuck with me while I walked you through the ongoing persistent challenges those with dyslexia can face from childhood into adulthood. Hopefully through this work you have gleaned some insights into the rocky road of being dyslexic; the yin and yang of our lives. How do you feel after learning about the struggles of those around you? What about their strengths - did you know these before? Let's look at the recommendations before we wrap up with some heart felt last words.

This research and work endeavours to advance the comprehension of the lived-experiences of adults with dyslexia, challenging established paradigms that suggest dyslexia has no bearing on adults. As a result, this work exposes incontestable disadvantages and obstacles enshrined across the ecological model for adults with dyslexia. The findings clearly indicate that these barriers are hindering the capacity of individuals with dyslexia to enjoy fulfilling and healthy lifestyles.

The creation of this research arose from my persistent frustration with the discrimination and lack of awareness that has characterised my personal and professional life. Through this work, I endeavour to explore and present the experiences of dyslexics as a reflection of my own lived-experiences. These subjective experiences have now been corroborated by the empirical findings of this thesis. This validation affirms that my struggles are not unique and that the lifelong impact of dyslexia on self-perception and feelings of low self-worth, incapability and difference are shared experiences. While more research is necessary, there is a pressing need for societal change towards a more accepting attitude towards neurodivergent disabilities such as dyslexia. So, what is the way forward?

10.1. THE WAY FORWARD

10.1.1. Community awareness and public health messaging

Dyslexia is a public health issue and, as such, Australian Federal and State Governments need to improve public awareness of dyslexia and its effects on individuals, their families and the broader community. Public awareness campaigns have been known to reduce smoking, enforce seatbelt wearing in cars, reduce the uptake of alcohol and other drugs. We are now seeing campaigns supporting autistic people and there is a place for increasing awareness and understanding of dyslexics, their needs and abilities.

10.1.2. Improved access to appropriate assessments and early intervention

National assessment standards including agreed upon terminology of dyslexia amongst industries is required to reduce the stigma, misunderstanding and poor community awareness of dyslexia, especially amongst health professionals and educational institutions. Aligning dyslexia with other neurodivergent conditions, such as autism, would ensure improved assessment and access to early interventions.

It is paramount that those in our community, especially children, can access timely diagnosis. The Australian Federal Government has a significant role to play in reducing societal inequalities faced by those with dyslexia. Policy and legislation must change if we are going to create equality for those with dyslexia. This could be improved by allocating an assessment item number for learning disabilities under the Medicare Benefits Scheme.

To support diagnosis and early interventions, individuals with dyslexia must be added to the National Disability Scheme. Research tells us that when early interventions are put in place, the impact of dyslexic difficulties can be reduced. This, in turn, improves education and employment outcomes and reduces the cost on the mental health system. Although dyslexia is the largest disability population, we also know there will be a sizeable percentage of dyslexics who do not require NDIS support. Dyslexia is a broad ranging spectrum condition and only those at the lower end would need ongoing support through the NDIS. A disability policy shift, that is inclusive of dyslexia within the National Disability Strategy, could increase success opportunities for dyslexic individuals by removing barriers, raising awareness of their strengths and weaknesses, and educating employers and educators about their needs. If the NDIS is not going to include dyslexia, government and experts should be coming together to look at other ways to ensure people get appropriate support, particularly to better support children and for those who are not in the workforce and can't access JobAccess.

10.1.3. mproved social and emotional well-being of dyslexic adults

Currently, there is a significant gap in the training provided to psychologists and mental health practitioners regarding dyslexia as a disability, particularly in understanding the profound and ongoing mental health challenges that individuals with dyslexia often encounter. These mental health issues are compounded by the lack of awareness and specialised support within the mental health profession. To address this gap, it is essential to integrate comprehensive training on dyslexia and its associated mental health effects into university curricula and professional development for psychologists, counsellors, and mental health practitioners. A focus on the dual diagnosis of dyslexia and co-occurring differences, alongside mental health conditions, should be embedded into educational practices, ensuring that future professionals are equipped to recognise and treat the complex needs of dyslexic individuals. This training would emphasise:

- Dyslexia as more than a learning difference, but as a disability with long-term emotional and psychological consequences.
- The link between dyslexia and mental health issues such as anxiety, depression and trauma, related to repeated academic failure or social exclusion.
- Neuro-affirming approaches that promote self-esteem and resilience in individuals with dyslexia.
- Evidence-based interventions tailored to support the mental health

and emotional well-being of people with dyslexia.

By embedding this into the educational framework of mental health courses, we can foster a new generation of practitioners who are better equipped to provide holistic, empathetic and effective care for those with dyslexia. This would lead to more accurate diagnoses, targeted interventions and improved mental health outcomes for individuals with dyslexia across all life stages.

10.1.4. Improve workplace practices through training

Workplaces must take a proactive, comprehensive approach to better understanding and supporting the needs of their dyslexic employees. This requires transformative change across the entire employment life-cycle, from recruitment and onboarding to career development, retention, and beyond. At its core, this transformation must focus on creating an inclusive, supportive environment that recognises both the unique challenges and strengths that dyslexic employees bring to the workplace. In a nutshell we need to see

- Dyslexic-friendly policies that support across the employment life-cycle.
- Training for Managers and Leadership, which is the cornerstone of this transformation. This includes identifying and mitigating unconscious bias that can affect how dyslexic employees are perceived and supported. Developing neuro-affirming language and communication styles and, most importantly, seeing the strengths of dyslexic employees rather than their differences.
- Implementing Best Practices across HR and Retention Strategies
- Adhering to and complying with federal, state and local legislation related to disability rights is not optional but obligatory. However,

compliance is just the baseline. To truly support dyslexic employees, organisations should be moving beyond legal obligations to work towards creating inclusive workplace cultures where everyone thrives.

Taking a proactive approach to supporting dyslexic employees means creating a workplace that is flexible, inclusive and legally compliant. Through policy reforms, improved inclusive practices, targeted training for leaders and managers, effective HR strategies, and adherence to legal frameworks, organisations can unlock the full potential of their dyslexic workforce. This not only improves retention and productivity but also drives innovation and a richer, more diverse organisational culture. Ultimately, investing in neurodivergence benefits everyone.

10.1.5. Streamlined and the states and government brought into alignment with access to health care, education and employment.

According to the Organisation for Economic Cooperation and Development (OECD) in 2017, Australia faces the risk of lagging behind other countries in terms of innovation and economic growth if it fails to invest in enhancing the literacy and numeracy skills of its population. This risk is particularly significant as other nations have made substantial investments in improving their citizens' literacy skills. Over the past three decades, the Federal Government has taken steps to streamline education standards, road safety and licensing, and aspects of the criminal code across the various states. We must look at doing the same for dyslexia as a disability. There is a pressing need for leadership that can guide and streamline dyslexia across education, employment and health with the states and territories to improve overall outcomes for individuals with dyslexia.

10.1.6. Increase in data collection and surveillance

It is evident that dyslexia is not adequately captured in government census statistics, and this must change, much like the recording of other neurodevelopmental conditions. Considering the high rates of dyslexia compared with other neurodevelopmental conditions, data needs to be collected and surveillance measures implemented to truly determine the significant impact that dyslexia has on individuals. This should include data collection through the Australian Census and the Australian Bureau of Statistics. This book should serve as a call to action to initiate this shift. By accurately understanding the true prevalence of dyslexia, governments should be compelled to do more by implementing appropriate provisions and policies in schools, higher education and the workplace, to better support those with dyslexia.

10.1.7. Future research

Based on the findings of this research, it is imperative that additional funding is allocated for further research to increase our understanding of the challenges faced by adults with dyslexia and to improve the quality of life for all Australians living with the condition. Currently, there is a glaring lack of research into dyslexia in adulthood within Australia; a gap that is both surprising and concerning given the profound impact dyslexia can have across all stages of life.

While much attention has been given to dyslexia in children and educational settings, there is a critical need to explore how dyslexia affects individuals as they transition into adulthood, enter the workforce and navigate complex social, emotional and cognitive demands. Adults with dyslexia often continue to experience significant barriers in professional and personal spheres, yet there is minimal data or research guiding effective support mechanisms tailored to their needs. Without targeted research, policymakers and practitioners are unable to implement effective solutions, leaving many dyslexic adults under-served. Addressing this research shortfall would not only provide deep-er insights into the lived-experiences of adults with dyslexia, but also empower governments, organisations and advocacy groups to develop better support systems, programs and policies aimed at improving the overall quality of life for this often-overlooked population. Expanding research in this area is essential for creating a more inclusive and equi-table society for all Australians living with dyslexia.

10.1.8. A proactive approach

The final recommendation is a proactive health promotion approach to dyslexia which is a public health issue. As mentioned earlier, being literate is a basic human right and if we take a proactive approach look-ing at protective factors that can enable dyslexic children to grow into strong, resilient, positive meaningful lives as adults, we need to start in the early years. I believe this is how we could start doing it ... today:

- working from a strength-based approach rather than focusing on their difficulties, to develop resilience and positive coping strategies that can be carried through into adulthood.
- encouraging and supporting friendships during childhood as a pro-tective factor against later relationship challenges.
- building self-advocacy and self-awareness skills from a young age
- providing dyslexia-specific education including mental health training across the education, high education and employment sectors.
- providing dyslexia training for allied health professionals who pro-vide counselling
- reviewing the decision to exclude dyslexia as a disability under the Medicare Benefits Scheme (MBS) and the National Disability In-

surance Scheme (NDIS), given dyslexia is classified as a disability under the Disability Discrimination Act.

- improving access to diagnosis and early intervention services by adding learning disabilities to the MBS and NDIS.
- Allied Health, teachers, support staff and the education sector should be training in dual diagnosis of dyslexia and mental health conditions.

That's a wrap

My mentor and I were talking about how I would wrap up this mammoth book of sadness and hope, and we talked about the golden threads that come together to create the people we are. 'The golden threads,' he said, 'the events throughout our lives that create the person we are today.' We spoke of the knock backs, the harsh words spoken to us, the name calling and the public humiliation we have faced. The tears of frustration, anger and feelings of not being good enough. Yet through all this there is something undeniable about dyslexics; it's our grit, resilience, determination and persistence. We are driven to get back up again, and again … to keep trying. Think about the dyslexics you know; those dyslexics finishing school and going on to TAFE or higher education, although school was so hard for them. All the working dyslexics climbing the career ladder, all the while 'passing' and 'masking' their dyslexia, putting in their own creative strategies to succeed. So many dyslexics create something that wasn't there before, out of necessity, because they didn't fit the mould or they saw a gap in the market to be filled. Think of the likes of Steve Jobs of Apple, or the birth of the *Dear Dyslexic podcast Show*, that turned into the *Dear Dyslexic Foundation,* the much need research and evidence about adulthood dyslexia. I know I'm not Steve Jobs but still,,, come on … there's been some great achievements!

All the setbacks and achievements - the golden threads of life - have shaped me into the person I am today. While I don't view dyslexia as a gift, and on most days not even as a strength, I can see how it has moulded me, enabling me to create and accomplish things I never would have imagined, things beyond my wildest dreams. If you had told me back in school that one day I'd be writing this book, building a global business, and most importantly, helping others, I would have laughed in disbelief. Yet here I am. And you, too, can become the person you aspire to be. Embrace the heartache, the highs, the lows, everything that has happened to you, and reflect on the golden threads that have woven together to form the tapestry of your life. As my mum's favourite Carole King song reminds me, we each have a unique and beautiful tapestry to tell.

So go forth and create a better world, not just for yourself, but for those around you, for those you work with, and lead with kindness. When we lead with kindness and empathy, we can change the world, and I hope through this research and the sharing of those with lived-experience you can create small changes, not just for those with dyslexia but for all you live and work with.

Glossary of Terms

Assistive Technology (AT): Any item, piece of equipment, software program, or product system that is used to increase, maintain or improve the functional capabilities of individuals with disabilities.

Ableism: Discrimination or social prejudice against individuals with disabilities, often based on the belief that typical abilities are superior. It manifests in attitudes, practices and policies that devalue or marginalise people with disabilities.

Autistic: Refers to individuals diagnosed with autism, a neurodevelopmental condition characterised by challenges with social interaction, communication, and repetitive behaviours.

ADHD: Attention Deficit Hyperactivity Disorder is a neurodevelopmental condition characterised by symptoms of inattention, hyperactivity and impulsivity that can affect an individual's ability to function effectively in daily life.

ADHDers: A term used by those who have ADHD

AuDHERs: A term that may refer to individuals who are autistic and ADHD.

Accessibility Features: Built-in functions of electronic devices and software that make them usable by people with disabilities. Examples include screen readers, closed captioning and voice recognition.

Bronfenbrenner Ecological Model: A theoretical framework developed by Urie Bronfenbrenner that emphasises the multiple layers of environmental influence on human development, including individual, family, community and societal factors.

Burnout: A state of physical and emotional exhaustion caused by prolonged stress and excessive demands, often leading to decreased productivity and job dissatisfaction.

Centrelink: Centrelink is a government agency in Australia that provides social security payments and services to individuals and families. It operates under the Department of Social Services and is managed by Services Australia.

Coach: A professional who provides guidance, support and training to individuals in various areas, such as career development or personal growth, helping them to achieve specific goals.

Co-occurring: Refers to the presence of two or more conditions in an individual, such as having both dyslexia and ADHD, which can complicate diagnosis and treatment.

Disability Discrimination Act:

Dyslexia: Individuals diagnosed with dyslexia; a specific learning disability that affects reading, writing and spelling abilities due to difficulties with phonological processing.

Dyslexic: A term used to describe those with dyslexia.

Dyspraxia: A developmental coordination condition that affects physical coordination and movement, leading to difficulties in performing tasks that require fine motor skills, such as writing or using tools.

Dysgraphia: A learning disability that affects writing abilities, characterised by difficulties with handwriting and organising thoughts on paper.

Dyscalculia: A specific learning disability that affects an individual's ability to understand and work with numbers, leading to difficulties in mathematical reasoning and calculations.

Diversity, Equality and Inclusion (DEI): A framework that promotes the fair treatment and full participation of all individuals, regardless of their background, identity or abilities, ensuring that diverse perspectives are valued and included.

Disclosure: The act of revealing one's disability or condition to others, which can be a significant step for individuals in seeking support and accommodations in various settings.

The Fair Work Act 2009: An Australian law that sets out the national workplace relations framework. It governs the rights and responsibilities of both employers and employees, ensuring fair and consistent treatment in the workplace. The Fair Work Act provides protections around minimum employment standards, workplace rights and dispute resolution.

Intersectionality: A concept that examines how various social identities (such as race, gender, sexuality and disability) intersect and create unique experiences of discrimination or privilege for individuals.

Identity First Language: A way of referring to individuals that emphasise their identity as part of a specific group, such as 'autistic person' or 'dyslexic individual,' reflecting a perspective that values the identity associated with the condition.

Learning Disability: A broad umbrella term that encompasses dyslexia, dysgraphia, dyscalculia and dyspraxia.

Job Demands-Resources Model: A theoretical framework that explains burnout as a result of an imbalance between job demands (physical, psychological, social or organisational aspects of the job that require sustained effort) and job resources (aspects of the job that help achieve work goals, reduce job demands, and stimulate personal growth).

Person First Language: A way of referring to individuals that emphasises their personhood before their condition, such as 'person with autism' or 'individual with dyslexia,' aiming to reduce stigma and promote respect.

JobAccess: An Australian government initiative that provides support and resources for people with disabilities to access employment opportunities, including funding for workplace modifications and training.

Mentor: An experienced and trusted advisor who provides guidance, support and encouragement to a less experienced individual, often in a professional or educational context.

Medical Model: A framework that views disability primarily as a medical issue, focusing on diagnosis, treatment and rehabilitation, often emphasising the individual's impairments rather than societal barriers.

Mental Health: A state of well-being that encompasses emotional, psychological and social factors, affecting how individuals think, feel and act, as well as how they handle stress and relate to others.

Medicare Benefits Scheme: The Medicare Benefits Scheme (MBS) is a key component of Australia's public healthcare system. It provides a list of medical services subsidised by the Australian government. Through the MBS, eligible Australian residents and certain overseas visitors can receive financial support for a range of healthcare services, including consultations with doctors and specialists, diagnostic tests and some surgical procedures.

MyGov: An Australian government online portal that provides a single, secure access point to a range of government services.

National Disability Scheme: The National Disability Insurance Scheme (NDIS) is an Australian government program designed to provide support and services to people with permanent and significant disabilities. Launched in 2013, the NDIS aims to improve the quality of life for individuals with disabilities by offering them greater choice and control over the support they receive.

Neurodiversity: The concept that neurological differences, such as those seen in autism and dyslexia, are a part of human diversity and should be recognised and respected, rather than pathologised.

Neurodivergence: A term that encompasses variations in the human brain and cognition, including conditions such as autism, ADHD, dyslexia and others, highlighting that these differences are natural and should be accepted.

Neuro-affirming Language: Language that recognises and respects neurodivergent individuals' experiences and identities, promoting acceptance and understanding of diverse neurological conditions.

NEAP – Neurodivergent Employment Assistance Program:

Human Resource (HR): The department within an organisation responsible for managing employee-related functions, including recruitment, training, performance management and employee relations.

Psychological Safety: A work environment where individuals feel safe to express their thoughts, ideas and concerns without fear of negative consequences, fostering open communication and collaboration.

Post-Traumatic Stress Disorder (PTSD): a mental health condition that can develop after an individual experiences or witnesses a traumatic event. It is characterised by a range of symptoms that can significantly impact daily life and functioning. Here is an overview of PTSD, its symptoms, causes, and treatment options.

People and Culture: A term often used interchangeably with Human Resources, focusing on fostering a positive organisational culture, employee engagement, and diversity and inclusion initiatives.

Social Model of Disability: A framework that views disability as a result of the interaction between individuals and societal barriers, emphasising the need for societal change to accommodate diverse abilities rather than focusing solely on individual impairments.

Screen Reader: A software application that identifies and interprets what is being displayed on a computer screen, then presents that information to the user via text-to-speech or a braille display. Commonly used by individuals who are blind or have low vision.

Text-to-Speech (TTS): A form of assistive technology that converts written text into spoken words. TTS software is used to read digital content aloud, enabling access for individuals with reading disabilities or visual impairments.

Voice Recognition: Software that translates spoken words into digital text, allowing users to control a computer or other device by voice rather than by mouse or keyboard. Useful for individuals with physical disabilities that impair their ability to type or use a mouse.

Universal Design: A design approach that aims to create products, environments and communications that are accessible and usable by all people, regardless of their age, ability, or status.

Universal Design for Learning (UDL): An educational framework that guides the design of flexible learning environments and materials to accommodate individual learning differences. UDL principles aim to make learning accessible for all students.

References

1. Milne, A.A. and E.H. Shepard, *Winnie-the-pooh*. 1992, England

2. Maguire, A., *Equality vs Equity* 2016, Interaction Institute for Social Change: Boston, Massachusetts.

3. Taggart, T., S. Stewart-Brown, and J. Parkinsi, *Warwick-Edinburgh Mental Well-being Scale (WEMWBS) User Guide*, 2, Editor. 2016, NHS Health Scotland: Edinburgh p. 62.

4. Taggart, F., S. Stewart-Brown, and J. Parkinson, *Warwick Edinburgh Mental Well-being Scale, User guide*. 2015, NHS, Health Scotland: Warwick Medical School, University of Warwick.

5. Bakker, A.B., E. Demerouti, and M.C. Euwema, *Job resources may buffer the impact of job demands on burnout.* Journal of occupational health psychology, 2005. **10**(2): p. 170.

6. Benson, W., *Job Demands Resources Model for Fostering Employee Engagement and Burnout* 2019: West Virgina.

7. Merriam-Webster Dictionary. *Dyslexia*. 2023 [cited 2023 19 May]; Available from: https://www.merriam-webster.com/dictionary/dyslexia#:~:text=Medical%20Definition-,dyslexia,in%20reading%2C%20spelling%2C%20and%20writing.

8. Collins Dictionary. *Defination of dyslexia*. 2023 [cited 2023 19 May]; Available from: https://www.collinsdictionary.com/dictio-

nary/english/dyslexia.

9. Hudson, J.P., *A Practical Guide to Congenital Developmental Disorders and Learning Difficulties* 2014, London: Routledge. 219.

10. Kirby, P., *Dyslexia debated, then and now: a historical perspective on the dyslexia debate.* Oxf Rev Educ, 2020. **46**(4): p. 472-486.

11. Eden, G.F., L. Flowers, and F. Wood, *Brain Imaging Studies of Reading and Reading Disability*, in *MIND Institute Lecture Series on Neurodevelopmental Disorders*, G.T.U. Center for the Study of Learning, Editor. 2015, University of California Television: California.

12. Dehaene, S. and G. Dehaene-Lambertz, *Is the brain prewired for letters?* Nat Neurosci, 2016. **19**(9): p. 1192-1193.

13. Dehaene, S., *How we learn : the new science of education and the brain*, ed. S. Dehaene. 2021: London : Penguin Books.

14. Lyon, G., S. Shaywitz, and B. Shaywitz, *A definition of dyslexia.* An Interdisciplinary Journal of The International Dyslexia Association, 2003. **53**(1): p. 1-14.

15. Yang, L., et al., *Prevalence of Developmental Dyslexia in Primary School Children: A Systematic Review and Meta-Analysis.* Brain Sci, 2022. **12**(2): p. 240.

16. Milberg, W., S. Blumstein, and B. Dworetzky, *Phonological processing and lexical access in aphasia.* Brain & Language, 1988. **34**(2): p. 279-93.

17. Gosvāmī, U., *Phonological skills and learning to read*, ed. P. Bryant. 1990, Hove: Hove : Lawrence Erlbaum.

18. Marshall, C.M., M.J. Snowling, and P.J. Bailey, *Rapid Auditory Processing and Phonological Ability in Normal Readers and Readers With Dyslexia.* J Speech Lang Hear Res, 2001. **44**(4): p. 925-940.

19. Knoop-van Campen, C.A.N., P.C.J. Segers, and L.T.W. Verhoeven, *How phonological awareness mediates the relation between work-*

ing memory and word reading efficiency in children with dyslexia. Dyslexia, 2018. **24**(2): p. 156-169.

20. Shaywitz, S.E. and B.A. Shaywitz, *Psychopathology of dyslexia and reading disorders.* 2013.

21. Pensettie, D. *What Is Specific Learning Disorder?* 2018 [cited 2020 21 April]; Available from: https://www.psychiatry.org/patients-families/specific-learning-disorder/what-is-specific-learning-disorder.

22. Berent, I., *On the Origins of Phonology.* Current Directions in Psychological Science : A Journal of the American Psychological Society, 2017. **26**(2): p. 132-139.

23. Snowling, J.M. and E.M. Hayiou-Thomas, *The Dyslexia Spectrum: Continuities Between Reading, Speech, and Language Impairments.* Topics in Language Disorders, 2006. **26**(2): p. 110-126.

24. Jordan, J.-A., G. McGladdery, and K. Dyer, *Dyslexia in Higher Education: Implications for Maths Anxiety, Statistics Anxiety and Psychological Well-being.* Dyslexia, 2014. **20**(3): p. 225-40.

25. Marks, R.A., et al., *Neurocognitive mechanisms of co-occurring math difficulties in dyslexia: Differences in executive function and visuospatial processing.* Developmental science, 2024. **27**(2): p. e13443-n/a.

26. Brosnan, M., et al., *Executive functioning in adults and children with developmental dyslexia.* Neuropsychologia, 2002. **40**(12): p. 2144-2155.

27. Lonergan, A., et al., *A meta-analysis of executive functioning in dyslexia with consideration of the impact of comorbid ADHD.* Journal of Cognitive Psychology, 2019. **31**(7): p. 725-749.

28. Leveroy, D.C., *Enabling performance: dyslexia, (dis)ability and 'reasonable adjustment'.* Theatre, dance and performance training, 2013. **4**(1): p. 87-101.

29. Waterfield, J., *Dyslexia: Implications for Learning, Teaching and Support.* Planet (Plymouth), 2002. **6**(1): p. 22-24.

30. Reid, G., *Dyslexia: A Practitioner's Handbook.* 5th ed. 2016, London: Continuum International Publishing Group.

31. Smart, D., et al., *Consequences of childhood reading difficulties and behaviour problems for educational achievement and employment in early adulthood.* British Journal of Educational Psychology, 2017. **87**(2): p. 288-308.

32. Boyes, M.E., et al., *Why are reading difficulties associated with mental health problems?.* Dyslexia (Chichester, England), 2016. **22**(3): p. 22.

33. Willcutt, E.G., et al., *Longitudinal study of reading disability and attention-deficit/hyperactivity disorder: Implications for education. [References].* 2007: Mind, Brain, and Education. Vol.1(4), 2007, pp. 181-192.

34. Richards, M., et al., *Long-term affective disorder in people with mild learning disability.* Br J Psychiatry, 2001. **179**(6): p. 523-527.

35. Macdonald, S.J., *"Journey's end": statistical pathways into offending for adults with specific learning difficulties.* Journal of learning disabilities and offending behaviour, 2012. **3**(2): p. 85-97.

36. Broidy, L.M., et al., *Developmental Trajectories of Childhood Disruptive Behaviors and Adolescent Delinquency: A Six-Site, Cross-National Study.* Developmental psychology, 2003. **39**(2): p. 222-245.

37. Chen, C.-C., F.J. Symons, and A.J. Reynolds, *Prospective Analyses of Childhood Factors and Antisocial Behavior for Students with High-Incidence Disabilities.* Behav Disord, 2011. **37**(1): p. 5-18.

38. Samuelsson, S., B. Herkner, and I. Lundberg, *Reading and Writing Difficulties Among Prison Inmates: A Matter of Experiential Factors Rather Than Dyslexic Problems.* Scientific studies of reading, 2003. 7(1): p. 53-73.

39. Caire, L., *Speech Pathology in Youth (Justice) Custodial Education Project Report*. 2013, The Speech Pathology Association of Australia Limited: Mlebourne. p. 56.

40. Caire, L., *Speech Pathology in Youth (Justice) Custodial Education Project Report*. 2013, The Speech Pathology Association of Australia Limited: Melbourne:.

41. Ankney, D., *Correlation Between Dyslexia and Criminal Behavior First Step Act to Require Screening, Treatment*. Prison Legal News, 2019. **30**(8): p. 30.

42. Hudson, R.F., L. High, and S. Al Otaiba, *Dyslexia and the Brain: What Does Current Research Tell Us?* The Reading teacher, 2007. **60**(6): p. 506-515.

43. Peterson, R. and B. Pennington, *Developmental dyslexia*. Lancet, 2012. **379**(9830): p. 1997-2007.

44. Maisog, J.M., et al., *A Meta-analysis of Functional Neuroimaging Studies of Dyslexia*. Ann N Y Acad Sci, 2008. **1145**(1): p. 237-259.

45. Berlingeri, M., et al., *Nouns and verbs in the brain: Grammatical class and task specific effects as revealed by fMRI*. Cogn Neuropsychol, 2008. **25**(4): p. 528-558.

46. Siegel, L.S., *IQ Is Irrelevant to the Definition of Learning Disabilities*. J Learn Disabil, 1989. **22**(8): p. 469-478.

47. Aaron, P.G., M. Joshi, and K.A. Williams, *Not all reading disabilities are alike*. Journal of Learning Disabilities, 1999. **32**(2): p. 120-137.

48. Goldstein, S., *Learning and Attention Disorders in Adolescence and Adulthood Assessment and Treatment*. 2nd ed.. ed, ed. J.A. Naglieri, M. DeVries, and S. Goldstein. 2011, Hoboken: Hoboken : John Wiley & Sons, Inc.

49. van Bergen, E., et al., *Child and parental literacy levels within fam-*

ilies with a history of dyslexia. J Child Psychol Psychiatry, 2012. **53**(1): p. 28-36.

50. Fisher, S.E. and J.C. DeFries, *Developmental dyslexia: genetic dissection of a complex cognitive trait.* Nature reviews. Neuroscience, 2002. **3**(10): p. 767-780.

51. Snowling, M.J., A. Gallagher, and U. Frith, *Family Risk of Dyslexia Is Continuous: Individual Differences in the Precursors of Reading Skill.* Child Development, 2003. **74**(2): p. 358-373.

52. Berninger, V.W., et al., *Writing problems in developmental dyslexia: Under-recognized and under-treated.(Report).* Journal of School Psychology, 2008. **46**(1): p. 1.

53. Grigorenko, E.L., et al., *Continuing the search for dyslexia genes on 6p.* American Journal of Medical Genetics. Part B, Neuropsychiatric Genetics: the Official Publication of the International Society of Psychiatric Genetics, 2003. **118B**(1): p. 89-98.

54. Brimo, K., et al., *The co-occurrence of neurodevelopmental problems in dyslexia.* Dyslexia, 2021. **27**(3): p. 277-293.

55. Pennington, B.F. and S.D. Smith, *Genetic influences on learning disabilities and speech and language disorders.* Child Development, 1983. **54**(2): p. 369-87.

56. Shanahan, L., et al., *Child-, adolescent- and young adult-onset depressions: differential risk factors in development?* Psychol Med, 2011. **41**(11): p. 2265-2274.

57. Kjersten, J., *Understanding and working with dyslexia in individual and couple therapy: Implications for counsellors and psychotherapists.* New Zealand Journal of Counselling, 2017. **37**: p. 1.

58. Livingston, E.M., L.S. Siegel, and U. Ribary, *Developmental dyslexia: emotional impact and consequences.* Australian Journal of Learning Difficulties, 2018. **23**(2): p. 107-135.

59. Wagner, R.K., et al., *The Prevalence of Dyslexia: A New Ap-*

proach to Its Estimation. Journal of learning disabilities, 2020: p. 22219420920377-22219420920377.

60. Kita, Y., F. Ashizawa, and M. Inagaki, *Prevalence estimates of neurodevelopmental disorders in Japan: A community sample questionnaire study.* Psychiatry Clin Neurosci, 2020. **74**(2): p. 118-123.

61. Ashraf, F. and N. Najam, *An epidemiological study of prevalence and comorbidity of non-clinical Dyslexia, Dysgraphia and Dyscalculia symptoms in Public and Private Schools of Pakistan.* Pak J Med Sci, 2020. **36**(7): p. 1659-1663.

62. Australia, E.S. *Nationally National Consistent Collection of Data of School Students with Disabilities.* 2022 [cited 2023 11 May].

63. Hendrickx, S., *The adolescent and adult neuro-diversity handbook : Asperger's syndrome, ADHD, dyslexia, dyspraxia and related conditions,* ed. ProQuest. 2010, London

Philadelphia: London

Philadelphia : Jessica Kingsley Publishers.

64. Pham, A. and A. Riviere, *Specific Learning Disorders and ADHD: Current Issues in Diagnosis Across Clinical and Educational Settings.* Current Psychiatry Reports, 2015. **17**(6): p. 1-7.

65. Russell, G., *Co-Occurrence of Developmental Disorders: Children Who Share Symptoms of Autism, Dyslexia and Attention Deficit Hyperactivity Disorder,* in *Recent Advances in Autism Spectrum Disorders,* M. Fitzgerald, Editor. 2013, s.l. : IntechOpen. p. 361-379.

66. Yeo, D., *Dyslexia, dyspraxia and mathematics.* Dyslexia, dyspraxia & mathematics, ed. I. Wiley. 2003, London: London : Whurr.

67. Bradshaw, A.R., et al., *Profile of language abilities in a sample of adults with developmental disorders.* Dyslexia, 2021. **27**(1): p. 3-28.

68. Haberstroh, S. and G. Schulte-Korne, *The Diagnosis and Treatment of Dyscalculia.* Deutsches Arzteblatt International, 2019. **116**(7): p. 107-114.

69. Wilson, A.J., et al., *Dyscalculia and dyslexia in adults: Cognitive bases of comorbidity.* Learning and Individual Differences, 2015. **37**: p. 118.

70. Butterworth, B., *Dyscalculia : from science to education.* 2019: London : Routledge.

71. Kucian, K. and M.v. Aster, *Developmental dyscalculia.* Eur J Pediatr, 2015. **174**(1): p. 1-13.

72. Willcutt, E.G., et al., *Comorbidity Between Reading Disability and Math Disability: Concurrent Psychopathology, Functional Impairment, and Neuropsychological Functioning.* J Learn Disabil, 2013. **46**(6): p. 500-516.

73. McBride, C., *Coping with dyslexia, dysgraphia and ADHD : A global perspective.* 2019, London: Routledge. p. 54-242.

74. McCloskey, M. and B. Rapp, *Developmental dysgraphia: An overview and framework for research.* Cogn Neuropsychol, 2017. **34**(3-4): p. 65-82.

75. Döhla, D. and S. Heim, *Developmental Dyslexia and Dysgraphia: What can We Learn from the One About the Other?* Front Psychol, 2015. **6**: p. 2045-2045.

76. Drotár, P. and M. Dobeš, *Dysgraphia detection through machine learning.* Sci Rep, 2020. **10**(1): p. 21541-21541.

77. Berninger, V.W. and D. Amtmann, *Preventing written expression disabilities through early and continuing assessment and intervention for handwriting and/or spelling problems: Research into practice,* in *Handbook of learning disabilities.* 2003, The Guilford Press: New York, NY, US. p. 345-363.

78. Kirby, A., D. Sugden, and C. Purcell, *Diagnosing developmental coordination disorders.* Arch Dis Child, 2014. **99**(3): p. 292-296.

79. Kirby, A., et al., *Dyslexia and developmental co-ordination disorder in further and higher education-similarities and differences. Does the*

'label' influence the support given? Dyslexia: the Journal of the British Dyslexia Association, 2008. **14**(3): p. 197-213.

80. Governement, A., *Draft National Autism Strategy*. 2024: Canberra.

81. Valkanova, V., F. Rhodes, and C.L. Allan, *Diagnosis and management of autism in adults*. Practitioner, 2013. **257**(1761): p. 13-6, 2-3.

82. Frith, U., *Autism and Dyslexia: A Glance Over 25 Years of Research*. Perspectives on psychological science, 2013. **8**(6): p. 670-672.

83. Newbury, D.F., D.V. Bishop, and A.P. Monaco, *Genetic influences on language impairment and phonological short-term memory*. Trends in Cognitive Sciences, 2005. **9**(11): p. 528-34.

84. Bishop, D.V.M., *The interface between genetics and psychology: lessons from developmental dyslexia*. Proc Biol Sci, 2015. **282**(1806): p. 20143139-20143139.

85. Oliveira, C.M., A.P. Vale, and J.M. Thomson, *The relationship between developmental language disorder and dyslexia in European Portuguese school-aged children*. J Clin Exp Neuropsychol, 2021. **43**(1): p. 46-65.

86. Snowling, M.J., et al., *Developmental Outcomes for Children at High Risk of Dyslexia and Children With Developmental Language Disorder*. Child Dev, 2019. **90**(5): p. e548-e564.

87. Catts, H.W., et al., *Are Specific Language Impairment and Dyslexia Distinct Disorders?* J Speech Lang Hear Res, 2005. **48**(6): p. 1378-1396.

88. McArthur, G.M., et al., *On the "Specifics" of Specific Reading Disability and Specific Language Impairment*. J Child Psychol Psychiatry, 2000. **41**(7): p. 869-874.

89. Price, K.M., et al., *Language Difficulties in School-Age Children With Developmental Dyslexia*. J Learn Disabil, 2022. **55**(3): p.

200-212.

90. Lawrence, D., et al., *The Mental Health of Children and Adolescents: Report on the second Child and Adolescent Survey of Mental Health and Wellbeing.*, D.o. Health, Editor. 2015, Australian Commonwealth: Canberra: .

91. Tully, L.A., et al., *A national child mental health literacy initiative is needed to reduce childhood mental health disorders.* . Australian & New Zealand Journal of Psychiatry, 2019. **53**(4): p. 4.

92. Nishida, A., M. Richards, and M. Stafford, *Prospective associations between adolescent mental health problems and positive mental wellbeing in early old age.(Report).* Child and Adolescent Psychiatry and Mental Health, 2016. **10**(1).

93. Alexander-Passe, N., *Dyslexia, traumatic schooling and career success: investigating the motivations of why many individuals with developmental dyslexia are successful despite experiencing traumatic schooling.* 2018, University of Sunderland: Sunderland. p. 376.

94. Leitao, S., et al., *Exploring the impact of living with dyslexia: The perspectives of children and their parents.* Int J Speech Lang Pathol, 2017. **19**(3): p. 322-334.

95. Alexander-Passe, N., *How children with dyslexia experience school: Developing an instrument to measure coping, self-esteem and depression.* 2020: Dissertation Abstracts International Section A: Humanities and Social Sciences. Vol.81(2-A),2020, pp. No Pagination Specified.

96. Zakopoulou, V., et al., *Specific learning difficulties: A retrospective study of their co morbidity and continuity as early indicators of mental disorders. [References].* 2014: Research in Developmental Disabilities. Vol.35(12), 2014, pp. 3496-3507.

97. McNulty, M.A., *Dyslexia and the Life Course.* Journal of Learning Disabilities, 2003. **36**(4): p. 363-381.

98. Wissell, S., L. Karimi, and T. Serry, *Adults with dyslexia: A snapshot of the demands on adulthood in Australia*. Australian journal of learning difficulties, 2021: p. 1-14.

99. Nelson, J.M. and S.W. Liebel, *Socially desirable responding and college students with dyslexia: Implications for the assessment of anxiety and depression. [References]*. 2018: Dyslexia: An International Journal of Research and Practice. Vol.24(1), 2018, pp. 44-58.

100. Alexander-Passe, N., *Dyslexia: Investigating Self-Harm and Suicidal Thoughts/Attempts as a Coping Strategy*. Journal of Psychology & Psychotherapy, 2015. **5**(6): p. 11.

101. Brunelle, K., S. Abdulle, and K.M. Gorey, *Anxiety and Depression Among Socioeconomically Vulnerable Students with Learning Disabilities: Exploratory Meta-analysis*. Child & adolescent social work journal, 2020. **37**(4): p. 359-367.

102. Alexander-Passe, N., *Dyslexia and depression: The hidden sorrow: An investigation of cause and effect*. Psychiatry - Theory, applications and treatments. 2012, New York: Novinka/Nova Science Publishers. 349.

103. Wilson, A., et al., *The Mental Health of Canadians With Self-Reported Learning Disabilities*. J Learn Disabil, 2009. **42**(1): p. 24-40.

104. Fuller-Thomson, E., S.Z. Carroll, and W. Yang, *Suicide Attempts among Individuals with Specific Learning Disorders: An Underrecognized Issue*. Journal of Learning Disabilities, 2018. **51**(3): p. 283-292.

105. Mental Health Foundation. *The cost of diagnosed mental health conditions: statistics*. 2023 [cited 2024 1 August]; Available from: https://www.mentalhealth.org.uk/explore-mental-health/mental-health-statistics/cost-diagnosed-mental-health-conditions-statistics#:~:text=The%20global%20cost%20of%20diagnosed%20

mental%20health%20conditions&text=Untreated%20m-
ental%20health%20problems%20account,of%20mortality%20
and%20morbidity%20globally.

106. Huda, A.S., *The medical model in mental health : an explanation and evaluation.* 2019: Oxford, England : Oxford University Press.

107. Serry, T.A. and L. Hammond, *What's in a word? Australian experts' knowledge, views and experiences using the term dyslexia.* Australian journal of learning difficulties, 2015. **20**(2): p. 143-161.

108. Luria, G., Y. Kalish, and M. Weinstein, *Learning disability and leadership: Becoming an effective leader.* J. Organiz. Behav, 2014. **35**(6): p. 747-761.

109. Mody, M. and E.R. Silliman, *Brain, Behaviour and Learing in Language and Reading Disorders*, C. Addison Stone, Editor. 2008, Guilford Press: NewYork. p. 103.

110. Beetham, J. and L. Okhai, *Workplace dyslexia & specific learning difficulties—productivity, engagement and well-being.* Open Journal of Social Sciences, 2017. **05**(06): p. 56-78.

111. Bond, J., *A comparative study of education policy in Scotland (United Kingdom) and New South Wales (Australia): the impact of two contrasting legislative and policy approaches on secondary students with dyslexia,*, in *College of Education, Psychology and Social Work.* 2021, Flinder's University: Bedford Park, South Australia. p. 250.

112. Snowling, C.T. Hulme, and K. Nation, *Defining and understanding dyslexia: past, present and future.* Oxf Rev Educ, 2020. **46**(4): p. 501-513.

113. American Psychiatric Association, *Learning Disorders*, in *Diagnostic and statistical manual of mental disorders (5th ed.).* 2013.

114. Glazzard, J. and K. Dale, *Trainee teachers with dyslexia: personal narratives of resilience.* Journal of Research in Special Educational Needs, 2013. **13**(1): p. 26-37.

115. Frolov, L. and M. Schaepper. *Diagnostic and Statistical Manual of Mental Disorders* What is a Specific Learning Disorders 2013 2021 [cited 2021 22 November]; 5:[Available from: https://www.psychiatry.org/patients-families/specific-learning-disorder/what-is-specific-learning-disorder.

116. Commonwealth of Australia, *Australia: Act No. 135 of 1992, Disability Discrimination Act 1992*. 1992, National Legislative Bodies / National Authorities: Canberra.

117. Education, D.o. *Understanding types of learning difficulty.* 2022 [cited 2023 11 April]; Available from: education.vic.gov.au/school/teachers/teachingresources/discipline/english/reading/Pages/understandings.aspx.

118. Moll, K., et al., *Specific learning disorder: prevalence and gender differences.* PLoS One, 2014. **9**(7): p. e103537-e103537.

119. World Health Organization. *International classification of diseases, 11th revision.* 2020 [cited 2022 8 August]; Available from: https://icd.who.int/en.

120. Commonwealth of Australia, *Fair Work Act* in *28*. 2009: Canberra. p. 585.

121. Commonwealth of Australia, *Equal Opportunity ACT 2010*. 2010: Canberra. p. 159.

122. Macdonald, S.J., *Towards a social reality of dyslexia.* British Journal of Learning Disabilities, 2010. **38**: p. 9.

123. Al-Yagon, M., et al., *The Proposed Changes for DSM-5 for SLD and ADHD : International Perspectives : Australia, Germany, Greece, India, Israel, Italy, Spain, Taiwan, United Kingdom, and United States.* J Learn Disabil, 2013. **46**(1): p. 58-72.

124. Owens, J., *Exploring the critiques of the social model of disability: the transformative possibility of Arendt's notion of power.* Sociol Health Illn, 2015. **37**(3): p. 385-403.

125. Hyde, M., *Exploring Disability: A Sociological Introduction. Colin Barnes, Geof Mercer and Tom Shakespeare. Cambridge: Polity, 1999, £49.50 (£14.95 pbk), 280 pp. (ISBN: 0-7456-1478-7).* Sociology, 2001. **35**(1): p. 219-258.

126. Shakespeare, T. and N. Watson, *Beyond Models: Understanding the Complexity of Disabled People's Lives.*, in *New Directions in the Sociology of Chronic and Disabling Conditions*, S.S.e. Scambler G., Editor. 2010, Palgrave Macmillan: London. p. 57-76.

127. Tregaskis, C., *Social Model Theory: The story so far.* Disability & society, 2002. **17**(4): p. 457-470.

128. Glazzard, J. and K. Dale, *'It Takes Me Half a Bottle of Whisky to Get through One of Your Assignments': Exploring One Teacher Educator's Personal Experiences of Dyslexia.* Dyslexia, 2015. **21**(2): p. 177-192.

129. Chappell, A.L., D. Goodley, and R. Lawthom, *Making connections: the relevance of the social model of disability for people with learning difficulties.* British journal of learning disabilities, 2001. **29**(2): p. 45-50.

130. Anastasiou, D. and J.M. Kauffman, *The Social Model of Disability: Dichotomy between Impairment and Disability.* J Med Philos, 2013. **38**(4): p. 441-459.

131. Denhart, H., *Deconstructing Barriers: Perceptions of Students Labeled With Learning Disabilities in Higher Education.* J Learn Disabil, 2008. **41**(6): p. 483-497.

132. Hughes, R., *The social model of disability.* British Journal of Healthcare Assistants, 2010. **4**(10): p. 508-511.

133. Macdonald, S.J., *Windows of reflection: conceptualizing dyslexia using the social model of disability.* Dyslexia, 2009. **15**(4): p. 347-362.

134. Riddick, B., *An Examination of the Relationship Between Labelling*

and Stigmatisation with Special Reference to Dyslexia. Disability & Society, 2000. **15**(4): p. 653-667.

135. Goodley, D., *'Learning Difficulties', the Social Model of Disability and Impairment: Challenging epistemologies.* Disability & society, 2001. **16**(2): p. 207-231.

136. Elftorp, P. and L. Hearne, *Understanding guidance counselling needs of adults with dyslexia through the lens of a critical-recognitive social justice perspective and a biopsychosocial model of disability.* Journal of the National Institute for Career Education and Counselling, 2020. **45**(1): p. 24-33.

137. Riddick, B., *Dyslexia and inclusion: Time for a social model of disability perspective?* International studies in sociology of education, 2001. **11**(3): p. 223-236.

138. Alexander-Passe, N., *Should 'developmental dyslexia' be understood as a disability or a difference?* Asia Pacific Journal of Developmental Differences, 2018. **5**: p. 247-271.

139. Alexander-Passe, *The dyslexia experience: difference, disclosure, labelling, discrimination and stigma.* Asia Pacific Journal of Developmental Differences, 2015. **2**(2): p. 33.

140. Walker, N., *NEUROQUEER HERESIES:Notes on the Neurodiversity Paradigm, Autistic Empowerment, and Postnormal Possibilities.* 2021, California: Autonomous press

141. Milton, D., *The Neurodiversity Reader: Exploring concepts, lived experiences and implication for practice.* 2020, West Sussex: Pavilion Publishing and Media.

142. Singer, J., *Neurodiversity: The birth of an idea.* 2016: Kindle eBook.

143. Jetha, A., et al., *Work-focused interventions that promote the labour market transition of young adults with chronic disabling health conditions: a systematic review.* Occupational & Environmental Med-

icine, 2019. **76**(3): p. 189-198.

144. Moody, S., *Dyslexia and employment : a guide for assessors, trainers and managers*. 2009: West Sussex, England : Wiley-Blackwell.

145. Wissell, S., et al., *"I hate calling it a disability": Exploring how labels impact adults with dyslexia through an intersectional lens. Under review*. Neurodiversity Journal, 2024.

146. Bronfenbrenner, U., *Developmental Research, Public Policy, and the Ecology of Childhood*. Child development, 1974. **45**(1): p. 1-5.

147. Bronfenbrenner, U., *Toward an experimental ecology of human development*. The American psychologist, 1977. **32**(7): p. 513-531.

148. Bronfenbrenner, U. and G.W. Evans, *Developmental Science in the 21st Century: Emerging Questions, Theoretical Models, Research Designs and Empirical Findings*. Social development (Oxford, England), 2000. **9**(1): p. 115-125.

149. Carbado, D.W., et al., *INTERSECTIONALITY: Mapping the Movements of a Theory*. Du Bois review, 2013. **10**(2): p. 303-312.

150. Saxe, A., *The Theory of Intersectionality: A New Lens for Understanding the Barriers Faced by Autistic Women*. Canadian journal of disability studies, 2017. **6**(4): p. 153-178.

151. Goethals, T., S. De, E., and H. Geert Van, *Weaving Intersectionality into Disability Studies Research: Inclusion, Reflexivity and Anti-Essentialism*. DiGeSt. Journal of Diversity and Gender Studies, 2015. **2**(1-2): p. 75-94.

152. Pal, G.C., *Disability, Intersectionality and Deprivation: An Excluded Agenda*. Psychology and developing societies, 2011. **23**(2): p. 159-176.

153. Bronfenbrenner, U., *Ecology of Human Development Experiments by Nature and Design*, ed. ProQuest. 2009, Cambridge: Cambridge : Harvard University Press.

154. SPELD Victoria. *Assessment costs*. 2020 [cited 2020 27 January];

Available from: https://www.speldvic.org.au/assessments/.

155. Wissell, S., *Dyslexia -The hidden disability in the workplace*, in *School of Psychology and Public Health* 2023, La Trobe: Melbourne. p. 256.

156. Commonwealth of Australia. *Australia's Disability Strategy 2021– 2031*. 2021 [cited 2022 15 May]; 72]. Available from: https:// www.dss.gov.au/disability-and-carers/a-new-national-disability-strategy

157. Gerber, P.J., C.G. Batalo, and E.O. Achola, *Dyslexia and Learning Disabilities in Canada and the UK: The Impact of its Disability Employment Laws*. Dyslexia, 2012. **18**(3): p. 166-173.

158. Marshall, J.E., et al., *"What should I say to my employer… if anything?"- My disability disclosure dilemma*. International journal of educational management, 2020. **34**(7): p. 1105-1117.

159. Morris, D. and P. Turnbull, *A survey-based exploration of the impact of dyslexia on career progression of UK registered nurses*. Journal of Nursing Management, 2007. **15**(1): p. 97-106.

160. Sabat, I.E., et al., *Invisible Disabilities: Unique Strategies for Workplace Allies*. Ind. organ. psychol, 2014. **7**(2): p. 259-265.

161. Sheldon, J., *Problematizing Reflexivity, Validity, and Disclosure: Research by People with Disabilities About Disability*. Qualitative report, 2017. **22**(4): p. 984.

162. von Schrader, S., V. Malzer, and S. Bruyère, *Perspectives on Disability Disclosure: The Importance of Employer Practices and Workplace Climate*. Employee responsibilities and rights journal, 2014. **26**(4): p. 237-255.

163. Price, L., P.J. Gerber, and R. Mulligan, *The Americans with Disabilities Act and Adults with Learning Disabilities as Employees: The Realities of the Workplace*. Remedial and special education, 2003. **24**(6): p. 350-358.

164. Gerber, P.J. and L.A. Price, *Self-Disclosure in Adults with Learning Disabilities and Dyslexia: Complexities and Considerations*, in *Supporting Dyslexic Adults in Higher Education and the Workplace*, N. Brunswick, Editor. 2012, John Wiley & Sons, Ltd.: London. p. 136-148.

165. Stampoltzis, A., E. Tsitsou, and G. Papachristopoulos, *Attitudes and intentions of Greek teachers towards teaching pupils with dyslexia: An application of the theory of planned behaviour.* Dyslexia: the Journal of the British Dyslexia Association, 2018. **24**(2): p. 128-139.

166. Wadlington, E.M. and P.L. Wadlington, *What educators really believe about dyslexia.* Reading improvement, 2005. **42**(1).

167. Attoe, D.E. and E.A. Climie, *Miss. Diagnosis: A Systematic Review of ADHD in Adult Women.* Journal of attention disorders, 2023. **27**(7): p. 645-657.

168. Werkhoven, S., J.H. Anderson, and I.A.M. Robeyns, *Who benefits from diagnostic labels for developmental disorders?* Developmental medicine and child neurology, 2022. **64**(8): p. 944-949.

169. Services, D.o.S. *JobAccess: Driving Disability Employment* 2024 [cited 2024 21 May]; Available from: https://www.jobaccess.gov.au/home.

170. Brzykcy, A. and S. Boehm, *No such thing as a free ride: The impact of disability labels on relationship building at work.* Human relations (New York), 2022. **75**(4): p. 734-763.

171. Gibson, B.E., *Worlding disability: Categorizations, labels, and the making of people.* AJOB neuroscience, 2019. **10**(2): p. 85-87.

172. Taylor, L.M., I.R. Hume, and N. Welsh, *Labelling and self-esteem: the impact of using specific vs. generic labels.* Educational Psychology, 2010. **30**(2): p. 191-202.

173. Wilson, R.B., et al., *Autistic women's experiences of self-compassion*

after receiving their diagnosis in adulthood. Autism : the international journal of research and practice, 2023. **27**(5): p. 1336-1347.

174. Sadusky, A., et al., *Diagnosing adults with dyslexia: Psychologists' experiences and practices.* Dyslexia (Chichester, England), 2021. **27**(4): p. 468-485.

175. Wechsler, D., *Wechsler Adult Intelligence Scale--Fourth Edition (WAIS-IV) APA PsycTests,* in *[Database record].* 2008, American Psychological Association: Washington.

176. Proger, B.B., *Test Review No. 18: Woodcock Reading Mastery Tests.* Journal of Special Education, 1975. **9**(4): p. 439-444.

177. Fletcher, J.M., et al., *Learning Disabilities: From Identification to Intervention, 2nd Edition.* 2 ed. 2019, New York: Guilford Publications.

178. Sadusky, A., et al., *Psychologists' diagnostic assessments of adults with dyslexia: an Australian-based survey study.* The educational and developmental psychologist, 2021. **ahead-of-print**(ahead-of-print): p. 1-10.

179. Bazen, L., et al., *Early and late diagnosed dyslexia in secondary school: Performance on literacy skills and cognitive correlates.* Dyslexia, 2020. **26**(4): p. 359-376.

180. Barbiero, C., et al., *The lost children: The underdiagnosis of dyslexia in Italy. A cross-sectional national study.* . PLoS ONE, 2019. **14**(1).

181. Torppa, M., et al., *Late-Emerging and Resolving Dyslexia: A Follow-Up Study from Age 3 to 14.* J Abnorm Child Psychol, 2015. **43**(7): p. 1389-1401.

182. Bent, C., *Factors associated with the age of diagnosis of autism in Australia: barriers and enablers to early identification policy responses,* in *College of Science, Health adn Engineering School of Psychology and Public Health, Autism Research Centre.* 2017, La Trobe Uni-

versity: Bundoora. p. 255.

183. Sullivan, E.L., et al., *Early identification of ADHD risk via infant temperament and emotion regulation: a pilot study.* Journal of Child Psychology and Psychiatry, 2015. **56**(9): p. 949-957.

184. Bond, J., et al., *Report to the Hon Bill Shorten, Parliamentary Secretary for Disabilities and Children's Services, from the Dyslexia Working Party.* 2010: Canberra.

185. British Dyslexia Association. *Who are our assessors?* 2020 [cited 2020 27 January]; Available from: https://www.bdadyslexia.org. uk/services/assessments/diagnostic-assessments/which-assessor.

186. Major, R. and J. Tetley, *Recognising, managing and supporting dyslexia beyond registration. The lived experiences of qualified nurses and nurse academics.* Nurse Education in Practice, 2019. **37**: p. 146-152.

187. Andresen, A. and M.-B. Monsrud, *Assessment of Dyslexia - Why, When, and with What?* Scandinavian journal of educational research, 2022. **66**(6): p. 1063-1075.

188. Waring, R. and R. Knight, *How should children with speech sound disorders be classified? A review and critical evaluation of current classification systems.* International Journal of Language & Communication Disorders, 2013. **48**(1): p. 25-40.

189. Australian Dyslexia Association. *Could it be dyslexia?* 2022 [cited 2022 17 July].

190. Richman, N., *Are you providing neurodiversity-affirming care?* 2022, Nicci Richman: Newcastle.

191. Bogart, K.R. and D.S. Dunn, *Ableism Special Issue Introduction.* Journal of social issues, 2019. **75**(3): p. 650-664.

192. Zeilinger, J. *6 Common Forms of Ableism we Need to Eliminate Immediately.* August 19 2015 [cited 2023 23.11.23].

193. Wissell, S., et al., *Leading Diverse Workforces: Perspectives from*

Managers and Employers about Dyslexic Employees in Australian Workplaces. International journal of environmental research and public health, 2022. **19**(19): p. 11991.

194. Eide, B. and F. Eide, *The Dyslexic Advantage: Unlocking the Hidden Potential of the Dyslexic Brain.* 2011: Penguin. 304.

195. Addison, R. and B. Cooke, *The value of dyslexia Dyslexic capability and organisations of the future.* 2019, Made by Dyslexia London. p. 26.

196. Dictionary.com. *Dyslexic thinking.* Dictonary 2024 [cited 2024 21 May]; Available from: https://www.dictionary.com/browse/dyslexic-thinking.

197. Dyslexia, M.B. *Dyslexic Thinking Campaign Film.* 2024 [cited 2024 21 May]; Available from: https://www.madebydyslexia.org/.

198. Moats, L. *Allegiance to the Facts: Best Approach for Students with Dyslexia.* 2016 [cited 2023 11 October]; Available from: https://dyslexiaida.org/allegiance-to-the-facts-best-approach-for-students-with-dyslexia/.

199. Hill Collins, P., *The Difference That Power Makes: Intersectionality and Participatory Democracy.* Investigaciones Feministas, 2017. **8**(1): p. 19-39.

200. Cohrdes, C. and E. Mauz, *Self-Efficacy and Emotional Stability Buffer Negative Effects of Adverse Childhood Experiences on Young Adult Health-Related Quality of Life.* J Adolesc Health, 2020. **67**(1): p. 93-100.

201. Daniel, S.S., et al., *Suicidality, School Dropout, and Reading Problems Among Adolescents.* J Learn Disabil, 2006. **39**(6): p. 507-514.

202. Westermair, A.L., et al., *All Unhappy Childhoods Are Unhappy in Their Own Way-Differential Impact of Dimensions of Adverse Childhood Experiences on Adult Mental Health and Health Behavior.* Front Psychiatry, 2018. **9**: p. 198-198.

203. Khasakhala, E., et al., *Comorbidity of mental health and autism spectrum disorder: perception of practitioners in management of their challenging behaviour.* International journal of developmental disabilities, 2023. **69**(3): p. 386-397.

204. Mitchelson, M., *Autism & ADHD in Girls and Women: Using Neurodiversity Affirming Therapy throughout the Lifespan.* 2024, PESIau: Chatswood.

205. Alexander-Passe, *Investigating Post-Traumatic Stress Disorder (PTSD) Triggered by the Experience of Dyslexia in Mainstream School Education?* Journal of Psychology & Psychotherapy 2015. **5**(6): p. 10.

206. Boyes, M.E., et al., *Correlates of externalising and internalising problems in children with dyslexia: An analysis of data from clinical casefiles.* Australian psychologist, 2020. **55**(1): p. 62-72.

207. Tanner, K., *Adult dyslexia and the 'conundrum of failure'.* Disability & Society, 2009. **24**(6): p. 785-797.

208. Caskey, J., P. Innes, and G.P. Lovell, *Making a Difference: Dyslexia and Social Identity in Educational Contexts.* Support for Learning, 2018. **33**(1): p. 73-88.

209. Maccullagh, L., *Participation and experiences of students with dyslexia in higher education: a literature review with an Australian focus.* Australian journal of learning difficulties, 2014. **19**(2): p. 93-111.

210. Serry, T.A. and F. Oberklaid, *Children with reading problems : Missed opportunities to make a difference.* The Australian journal of education, 2015. **59**(1): p. 22-34.

211. Maxwell, C., *Teacher education on dyslexia : An analysis of policy and practice in Australia and England.* Education, research and perspectives, 2019. **46**(2019): p. 1-19.

212. de Beer, J., et al., *Factors influencing work participation of adults*

with developmental dyslexia: a systematic review. BMC Public Health, 2014. **14**(1).

213. Kornblau, B.L., *Fieldwork education and students with disabilities: enter the Americans With Disabilities Act.* American Journal of Occupational Therapy, 1995. **49**(2): p. 139-45.

214. Lauder, K.M., *A critical examination of the evidence for effective reasonable adjustments for adults with attention deficit hyperactivity disorder in the workplace.* 2020, Birkbeck.

215. King, L., *Exploring student nurses' and their link lecturers' experiences of reasonable adjustments in clinical placement.* British Journal of Nursing, 2019. **28**(17): p. 1130-1134.

216. Gerber, P.J., et al., *Persisting Problems of Adults with Learning Disabilities: Self-Reported Comparisons From Their School-Age and Adult Years.* Journal of Learning Disabilities, 1990. **23**(9): p. 570-573.

217. Nelson, J.M. and N. Gregg, *Depression and anxiety among transitioning adolescents and college students with ADHD, dyslexia, or comorbid ADHD/dyslexia. [References].* 2012: Journal of Attention Disorders. Vol.16(3), 2012, pp. 244-254.

218. Nelson, J.M., W. Lindstrom, and P.A. Foels, *Test anxiety among college students with specific reading disability (dyslexia): Nonverbal ability and working memory as predictors. [References].* 2015: Journal of Learning Disabilities. Vol.48(4), 2015, pp. 422-432.

219. Friborg, O., et al., *Resilience in relation to personality and intelligence.* Int. J. Methods Psychiatr. Res, 2005. **14**(1): p. 29-42.

220. Hellendoorn, J. and W. Ruijssenaars, *Personal Experiences and Adjustment of Dutch Adults with Dyslexia.* Remedial and special education, 2000. **21**(4): p. 227-239.

221. Greenbaum, B., S. Graham, and W. Scales, *Adults with Learning Disabilities: Educational and Social Experiences during College.* Ex-

ceptional children, 1995. **61**(5): p. 460-471.

222. Stack-Cutler, H.L., R.K. Parrila, and M. Torppa, *Using a multidimensional measure of resilience to explain life satisfaction and academic achievement of adults with reading difficulties.* Journal of Learning Disabilities, 2015. **48**: p. 646-657.

223. Litner, B., V. Mann-Feder, and G. Guérard, *Narratives of success: Learning disabled students in university.* . Exceptionality Education Canada, 2005. **15**: p. 9-23.

224. Moore, T. and L. Carey, *Friendship formation in adults with learning disabilities: peer-mediated approaches to social skills development.* British Journal of Learning Disabilities, 2005. **33**(1): p. 23-26.

225. Weigel, L., et al., *Challenging behaviour and learning disabilities: the relationship between expressed emotion and staff attributions.* British Journal of Clinical Psychology, 2006. **45**(Pt 2): p. 205-16.

226. Stack-Cutler, H.L., *Examining resilience among university students with reading difficulties using internal and external protective factors.* 2017: Dissertation Abstracts International Section A: Humanities and Social Sciences. Vol.77(9-A(E)),2017, pp. No Pagination Specified.

227. Alexander-Passe, *The Experience of Being Married to a Dyslexic Adult.* Journal of Psychology & Psychotherapy, 2015. **5:6**: p. 12.

228. Ganz, J., *Learning Disabilities and Life Stories.* 2001. **36**: p. 245.

229. Nalavany, B.A. and L.W. Carawan, *Perceived Family Support and Self-Esteem: The Mediational Role of Emotional Experience in Adults with Dyslexia.* Dyslexia, 2012. **18**(1): p. 58-74.

230. Nalavany, B.A., L.W. Carawan, and R.A. Rennick, *Psychosocial Experiences Associated with Confirmed and Self-Identified Dyslexia: A Participant-Driven Concept Map of Adult Perspectives.* Journal of Learning Disabilities, 2011. **44**(1): p. 63-79.

231. Fernańdez-Alcántara, M., et al., *Feelings of loss and grief in par-*

ents of children diagnosed with autism spectrum disorder (ASD). Research in developmental disabilities, 2016. **55**: p. 312-321.

232. Gilliver, M., T.Y.C. Ching, and J. Sjahalam-King, *WHEN EXPECTATION MEETS EXPERIENCE: PARENTS' RECOLLECTIONS OF AND EXPERIENCES WITH A CHILD DIAGNOSED WITH HEARING LOSS SOON AFTER BIRTH.* International journal of audiology, 2013. **52**(2).

233. Bravo-Benítez, J., et al., *Grief Experiences in Family Caregivers of Children with Autism Spectrum Disorder (ASD).* International journal of environmental research and public health, 2019. **16**(23): p. 4821.

234. Fernández-Ávalos, M.I., et al., *Feeling of grief and loss in parental caregivers of adults diagnosed with intellectual disability.* Journal of applied research in intellectual disabilities, 2021. **34**(3): p. 712-723.

235. Denton, K., et al., *Parents' voices matter: A mixed-method study on the dyslexia diagnosis process.* Psychology in the schools, 2022. **59**(11): p. 2267-2286.

236. Carawan, L.W., B.A. Nalavany, and C. Jenkins, *Emotional experience with dyslexia and self-esteem: the protective role of perceived family support in late adulthood.* Aging & Mental Health, 2016. **20**(3): p. 284-294.

237. Thiagarajan, A. and N.A. Muhammad, *A Case Study on Sibling Relational Problem: Its Clinical Significance in Managing A Dyslexic Adolescent with Mild Depressive Disorder.* Jurnal sains kesihatan Malaysia, 2022. **20**(2): p. 35-40.

238. Alexander-Passe, N., *Dyslexics dating, marriage and parenthood.* 1st ed.. ed, ed. N. Alexander-Passe. 2012, New York: New York : Nova Science Publishers, Inc.

239. Trew, S., *Close Relationships Despite the Challenges: Sibling Rela-*

tionships and Autism. Journal of autism and developmental disorders, 2024.

240. Peasgood, T., et al., *The impact of ADHD on the health and well-being of ADHD children and their siblings*. European child & adolescent psychiatry, 2016. **25**(11): p. 1217-1231.

241. Polan, S., et al., *Siblings of autism : the challenge & the hope*. 2014, Grand Junction, CO : Listen 2 Kids Productions, LLC.

242. Hastings, R.P. and M.A. Petalas, *Self-reported behaviour problems and sibling relationship quality by siblings of children with autism spectrum disorder*. Child : care, health & development, 2014. **40**(6): p. 833-839.

243. Campbell, F., et al., *Early Childhood Investments Substantially Boost Adult Health*. Science, 2014. **343**(6178): p. 1478-1485.

244. Katz, S. and T. Calasanti, *Critical perspectives on successful aging: does it "appeal more than it illuminates"?* Gerontologist, 2015. **55**(1): p. 26-33.

245. Terras, M.M., L.C. Thompson, and H. Minnis, *Dyslexia and psycho-social functioning: an exploratory study of the role on self-esteem and understanding*. Dyslexia, 2009. **15**(4): p. 304-327.

246. Boetsch, E.A., P.A. Green, and B.F. Pennington, *Psychosocial correlates of dyslexia across the life span*. 1996: Development and Psychopathology. Vol.8(3), 1996, pp. 539-562.

247. Fogler, J.M. and R.A. Phelps, *Trauma, Autism, and Neurodevelopmental Disorders Integrating Research, Practice, and Policy*. 2018: Cham : Springer International Publishing : Imprint: Springer.

248. Thompson, R.A., *Stress and child development*. Future of Children, 2014. **24**(1): p. 41-59.

249. Haruvi-Lamdan, N., D. Horesh, and O. Golan, *PTSD and Autism Spectrum Disorder: Co-Morbidity, Gaps in Research, and Potential Shared Mechanisms*. Psychological trauma, 2018. **10**(3): p.

290-299.

250. Creamer, M., P. Burgess, and A.C. McFarlane, *Post-traumatic stress disorder: findings from the Australian National Survey of Mental Health and Well-being.* Psychological medicine, 2001. **31**(7): p. 1237-1247.

251. Stenner, A.J. and G.K. William, *Self-Concept Development in Young Children.* Phi Delta Kappan, 1976. **58**(4): p. 356-357.

252. Graham, D.M., *Speaking for Themselves: Ethnographic Interviews with Adults with Learning Disabilities* Journal of Reading, 1992. **36**(1): p. 74-75.

253. Olympia, P., *Dyslexia and self-concept: Seeking a dyslexic identity.* 2006, Leicester: Leicester: British Psychological Society. 202.

254. Humphrey, N. and P.M. Mullins, *Self-concept and self-esteem in developmental dyslexia.* Journal of research in special educational needs, 2002. **2**(2).

255. Australian Psychology Society, *Stress & wellbeing - how Australians are coping with life.* 2015, Australian Psychology Society: Melbourne. p. 43.

256. Wissell, S., et al., *"You Don't Look Dyslexic": Using the Job Demands-Resource Model of Burnout to Explore Employment Experiences of Australian Adults with Dyslexia.* International Journal of Environmental Research and Public Health, 2022. **19**(17): p. 10719.

257. Bartlett, D., S. Moody, and K. Kindersley, *Dyslexia in the workplace : an introductory guide.* 2nd ed.. ed, ed. S. Moody and K. Kindersley. 2010, Chichester Malden, MA: Wiley-Blackwell.

258. Hagan, B., *Dyslexia in the Workplace TUC Guides*, 3, Editor. 2014: England.

259. Major, R. and J. Tetley, *Effects of dyslexia on registered nurses in practice.* Nurse Education in Practice, 2019. **35**: p. 7-13.

260. Locke, R., et al., *Doctors with dyslexia: strategies and support.* Clin Teach, 2017. **14**(5): p. 355-359.

261. Le Cunff, A.L., E. Dommett, and V. Giampietro, *Neurophysiological measures and correlates of cognitive load in attention-deficit/ hyperactivity disorder (ADHD), autism spectrum disorder (ASD) and dyslexia: A scoping review and research recommendations.* The European journal of neuroscience, 2024. **59**(2): p. 256-282.

262. Sewell, J.L., L. Santhosh, and P.S. O'Sullivan, *How do attending physicians describe cognitive overload among their workplace learners?* Medical education, 2020. **54**(12): p. 1129-1136.

263. Jaeggi, S.M., et al., *On how high performers keep cool brains in situations of cognitive overload.* Cognitive, affective, & behavioral neuroscience, 2007. **7**(2): p. 75-89.

264. Jones, F., J. Hamilton, and N. Kargas, *Accessibility and affirmation in counselling: An exploration into neurodivergent clients' experiences.* Counselling and psychotherapy research, 2024.

265. Valeras, A., *"We don't have a box": Understanding Hidden Disability Identity Utilizing Narrative Research Methodology.* Disability Studies Quarterly, 2010. **30**(3/4).

266. Ernst and Young, *The value of dyslexia Dyslexic capability and organisations of the future.* 2019: London. p. 28.

267. Brewerton, P., *Using strengths to drive career success.* Strategic HR review, 2011. **10**(6): p. 5-10.

268. Xanthopoulou, D., et al., *The Role of Personal Resources in the Job Demands-Resources Model.* International journal of stress management, 2007. **14**(2): p. 121-141.

269. Burns, E., A.-M. Poikkeus, and M. Aro, *Resilience strategies employed by teachers with dyslexia working at tertiary education.* Teaching and Teacher Education, 2013. **34**: p. 77.

270. Leather, C., et al., *Cognitive functioning and work success in adults*

with dyslexia. Dyslexia: the Journal of the British Dyslexia Association, 2011. **17**(4): p. 327-38.

271. Goldberg, R.J., et al., *Predictors of Success in Individuals with Learning Disabilities: A Qualitative Analysis of a 20-Year Longitudinal Study.* Learning disabilities research and practice, 2003. **18**(4): p. 222-236.

272. Dyslexia, M.B., *The Intelligence 5.0, a new school of thought rethinking the intelligence needed in the Industry 5* 2024: U.K. p. 108.

273. Gignac, M.A.M., et al., *Does it matter what your reasons are when deciding to disclose (or not disclose) a disability at work? The association of workers' approach and avoidance goals with perceived positive and negative workplace outcomes.* J Occup Rehabil, 2021. **31**(3): p. 638-651.

274. McLoughlin, D., *Career development and indiviudals with dyslexia* Career Planning and Adult Development Journal, 2015. **31**(4): p. 10.

275. Morris, D. and P. Turnbull, *The disclosure of dyslexia in clinical practice: experiences of student nurses in the United Kingdom.* Nurse Education Today, 2007. **27**(1): p. 35-42.

276. Rose, J., *Independent review of the teaching of early reading: Final Report*, D.f.E.a. Skills, Editor. 2006: England.

277. Newlands, F., D. Shrewsbury, and J. Robson, *Foundation doctors and dyslexia: a qualitative study of their experiences and coping strategies.* Postgraduate Medical Journal, 2015. **91**(1073): p. 121-6.

278. Madaus, J.W., *Employment self-disclosure rates and rationales of university graduates with learning disabilities.* Journal of Learning Disabilities, 2008. **41**(4): p. 291-9.

279. Santuzzi, A.M., et al., *Invisible Disabilities: Unique Challenges for Employees and Organizations.* Ind. organ. psychol, 2014. **7**(2): p.

204-219.

280. Lemos, C.d., et al., *Awareness of developmental language disorder amongst workplace managers.* J Commun Disord, 2022. **95**: p. 106165-106165.

281. Australian Institute Health and Welfare. *Employment and unemployment.* 2022 [cited 2022 6 January]; Available from: https://www.aihw.gov.au/reports/australias-welfare/employment-trends.

282. Kirby, A. and H. Gibbon, *Dyslexia and Employment.* Perspectives on language and literacy, 2018. **44**(1): p. 27-31.

283. Maughan, B., M. Rutter, and W. Yule, *The Isle of Wight studies: the scope and scale of reading difficulties.* Oxford Review of Education, 2020. **46**(4): p. 10.

284. Maughan, B., et al., *Persistence of literacy problems: spelling in adolescence and at mid-life.* J Child Psychol Psychiatry, 2009. **50**(8): p. 893-901.

285. Macdonald, S.J. and L. Deacon, *Twice upon a time: Examining the effect socio-economic status has on the experience of dyslexia in the United Kingdom.* Dyslexia: the Journal of the British Dyslexia Association, 2019. **25**(1): p. 3-19.

286. Strawa, C. *Supporting young people experiencing disadvantage to secure work.* 2022 [cited 2024 4 Janaury]; Available from: https://aifs.gov.au/resources/short-articles/supporting-young-people-experiencing-disadvantage-secure-work#:~:text=Young%20people%20who%20are%20not,experiencing%20future%20long%2Dterm%20unemployment.

287. McKay, J. and J. Neal, *Diagnosis and disengagement: exploring the disjuncture between SEN policy and practice.* Journal of Research in Special Educational Needs, 2009. **9**(3): p. 164-172.

288. Telwatte, A., et al., *Workplace Accommodations for Employees With Disabilities: A Multilevel Model of Employer Decision-Making.* Re-

habil Psychol, 2017. **62**(1): p. 7-19.

289. Sheppard-Jones, K., et al., *Reframing workplace inclusion through the lens of universal design: Considerations for vocational rehabilitation professionals in the wake of COVID-19.* Journal of vocational rehabilitation, 2021. **54**(1): p. 71-79.

290. Finn, M., et al., *'If I'm just me, I doubt I'd get the job': A qualitative exploration of autistic people's experiences in job interviews.* Autism : the international journal of research and practice, 2023. **27**(7): p. 2086-2097.

291. McMillan, J.T., B. Listyg, and J. Cooper, *Neurodiversity and talent measurement: Revisiting the basics.* Industrial and organizational psychology, 2023. **16**(1): p. 31-35.

292. Flower, R.L., L.M. Dickens, and D. Hedley, *Barriers to Employment: Raters' Perceptions of Male Autistic and Non-Autistic Candidates During a Simulated Job Interview and the Impact of Diagnostic Disclosure.* Autism in adulthood, 2021. **3**(4): p. 300-309.

293. Safe Work Australia. *Mental health.* 2020 2020 [cited 2021 7 February]; Available from: https://www.safeworkaustralia.gov.au/topic/mental-health.

294. Aid, M.H.F. *Navigating burnout: Tips for mental health.* 2024 [cited 2024 3 August]; Available from: https://www.mhfa.com.au/navigating-burnout/.

295. UiPath, *Global Knowledge Worker Survey Insights into how knowledge workers are using GenAI and automation.* 2024: United State.

296. People at Work. *Helping to create psychologically healthy and safe workplaces.* 2024 [cited 2024 3 September]; Available from: https://www.peopleatwork.gov.au/.

297. People at Work. *Psychological health for small business.* 2024 [cited 2024 3 September].

298. Australia, S.W., *Managing psychosocial hazards at work Code of*

Practice. 2022: Canberra. p. 54.

299. World Health Organisation (WHO). *Burn-out an "occupational phenomenon"*. 2024 [cited 2024 3 August]; Available from: https://www.who.int/standards/classifications/frequently-asked-questions/burn-out-an-occupational-phenomenon#:~:text=%E2%80%9CBurn%2Dout%20is%20a%20syndrome,related%20to%20one's%20job%3B%20and.

300. Brauchli, R., et al., *Disentangling stability and change in job resources, job demands, and employee well-being — A three-wave study on the Job-Demands Resources model*. Journal of vocational behavior, 2013. **83**(2): p. 117-129.

301. Akkermans, J., et al., *The role of career competencies in the job demands - resources model*. Journal of vocational behavior, 2013. **83**(3): p. 356-366.

302. Xanthopoulou, D., et al., *Reciprocal relationships between job resources, personal resources, and work engagement*. Journal of vocational behavior, 2009. **74**(3): p. 235-244.

303. Jang, J., W. Jo, and J.S. Kim, *Can employee workplace mindfulness counteract the indirect effects of customer incivility on proactive service performance through work engagement? A moderated mediation model*. Journal of hospitality marketing & management, 2020. **29**(7): p. 812-829.

304. Van den Broeck, A., et al., *Not all job demands are equal: Differentiating job hindrances and job challenges in the Job Demands-Resources model*. European journal of work and organizational psychology, 2010. **19**(6): p. 735-759.

305. Schaufeli, W.B., *Applying the Job Demands-Resources Model : A 'how to' guide to measuring and tackling work engagement and burnout*. Organizational dynamics, 2017. **46**(2): p. 120.

306. Bakker, A.B. and E. Demerouti, *The Job Demands-Resources model:*

state of the art. Journal of managerial psychology, 2007. **22**(3): p. 309-328.

307. Feng, L.C., et al., *Job demands, job resources and safety outcomes: The roles of emotional exhaustion and safety compliance.* Accid Anal Prev, 2013. **51**: p. 243-251.

308. Bell, S., *Exploring support for dyslexic adults in the English workforce: lessons learnt from the story of an adult dyslexia group.* Support for Learning, 2009. **24**(2): p. 73-80.

309. Graham, L.J., *Inclusive education for the 21st century : theory, policy and practice.* Inclusive education for the twenty first century. 2020: Crows Nest, NSW : Allen & Unwin.

310. Nalavany, B.A., J.M. Logan, and L.W. Carawan, *The relationship between emotional experience with dyslexia and work self-efficacy among adults with dyslexia. [References].* 2018: Dyslexia: An International Journal of Research and Practice. Vol.24(1), 2018, pp. 17-32.

311. Deacon, L., S.J. Macdonald, and J. Donaghue, *"What's wrong with you, are you stupid?" Listening to the biographical narratives of adults with dyslexia in an age of 'inclusive' and 'anti-discriminatory' practice.* Disability & society, 2020: p. 1-21.

312. Wallace, J.E. and J. Lemaire, *Physician Coping Styles and Emotional Exhaustion.* Relations industrielles (Québec, Québec), 2013. **68**(2): p. 187-209.

313. Locke, R., et al., *Clinicians with dyslexia: a systematic review of effects and strategies.* Clin Teach, 2015. **12**(6): p. 394-398.

314. Shrewsbury, D., *Dyslexia in general practice education: considerations for recognition and support.* Education for Primary Care, 2016. **27**(4): p. 267-70.

315. Gerber, P.J., et al., *Beyond transition: a comparison of the employment experiences of American and Canadian adults with LD.* Journal of Learning Disabilities, 2004. **37**(4): p. 283-91.

316. Kreider, C.M., S. Medina, and M.R. Slamka, *Strategies for Coping with Time-Related and Productivity Challenges of Young People with Learning Disabilities and Attention-Deficit/Hyperactivity Disorder.* Children, 2019. **6**(2): p. 13.
317. McDowall, A., *Neurodiversity Coaching: A Psychological Approach to Supporting Neurodivergent Talent and Career Potential.* First edition.. ed, ed. N. Doyle. 2024: Milton Park, England: Routledge.

www.ingramcontent.com/pod-product-compliance
Lightning Source LLC
Chambersburg PA
CBHW031142020426
42333CB00013B/477